T0270905

This unique source of reference provides the first comprehensive guide to the adverse side effects of many commonly prescribed drugs on fertility and sexual health. More than 150 drugs are listed in this compilation, and the evidence linking them with infertility and sexual dysfunction is carefully reviewed. The volume is designed to provide a rapid source of reference to alert doctors and pharmacists to these hazardous side effects. The volume also includes an introductory account of the reproductive process and a review of the mechanisms by which these drugs can interfere with or inhibit reproduction. Another important theme of the volume is the effect of social and recreational drugs and environmental agents on reproductive health. This compilation will be an essential source of reference for doctors, pharmacists and other health care professionals.

Drug-induced infertility and sexual dysfunction

Drug-induced infertility and sexual dysfunction

Robert Forman

Susanna Gilmour-White

Nathalie Forman

Guy's and St Thomas' Hospitals, London

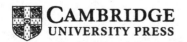
CAMBRIDGE
UNIVERSITY PRESS

Published by the Press Syndicate of the University of Cambridge
The Pitt Building, Trumpington Street, Cambridge CB2 1RP
40 West 20th Street, New York, NY 10011-4211 USA
10 Stamford Road, Oakleigh, Melbourne 3166, Australia

© Cambridge University Press 1996

First published 1996

A catalogue record for this book is available from the British Library

Library of Congress cataloguing in publication data

Forman, Robert.
    Drug induced infertility and sexual dysfunction / Robert Forman,
Susanna Gilmour-White, Nathalie Forman.
        p.   cm.
    ISBN 0 521 46563 X (hc)
        1. Generative organs – Effect of drugs on.   2. Drugs – Side effects.
3. Infertility.   4. Sexual disorders.   I. Gilmour-White, Susanna.
II. Forman, Nathalie.   III. Title.
    RC877.F67   1996
    616.6′9071–dc20   95-32836 CIP

ISBN 0 521 46563 X hardback

Transferred to digital printing 2003

Contents

Preface

The idea for this book originated from the professional frustration experienced by the authors in the face of apparently simple enquiries from patients or health care colleagues. Questions on the possibility that patients' fertility or sexual problems could be drug related resulted in extensive literature searches, discussions with pharmaceutical companies and, sometimes, contact with the Committee on Safety of Medicines. These endeavours generated a collection of academic papers requiring time-consuming analysis before a reply could be given.

The desirability for a comprehensive reference text which included much of this information in a readily accessible form was all too evident.

One of the difficulties in a project of this type is the source of data. We were only able to access information in the public domain. Two important sources of valuable data are not available to the public. These are the databases collated by the Committee on Safety of Medicines via the yellow card notification scheme and those held by pharmaceutical manufacturers. Manufacturers have a reporting obligation to notify the Committee on Safety of Medicines about serious or life-threatening adverse effects. Infertility and sexual dysfunction do not come into this category.

Academic journals are the major reference source for much of the information in this book. Adverse drug effects may be published as case reports, which can be useful early warnings of a potential problem but do not necessarily represent general experience. Controlled clinical trials of adverse reproductive effects are few and far between but have been included where available. Many drugs are given for diseases which can themselves affect reproductive function and this is highlighted in the relevant sections. Even when an association between drug consumption and reproductive dysfunction is present, confounding variables such as lifestyle and the use of other drugs etc. may prevent conclusions about causality.

An attempt has been made in this book to present to the reader the evidence available to date so that, when confronted with a clinical situation which could implicate a particular drug, an informed clinical judgement can be made quickly and easily.

Not all drugs affecting reproductive function are medically prescribed. Socially acceptable or recreational drugs have also been implicated, as have some drugs of abuse. We have included a chapter on these as a certain mythology surrounds many of these substances and patients do wish to know how their lifestyle may influence their sexual health. Also this is an area where good epidemiological studies have been performed.

The final chapter in this book is dedicated to environmental agents. Whilst not falling within the definition of the term drugs, many chemical and physical agents have been shown to provoke major degrees of reproductive disease. Public concern on these issues is increasing and a new science of reproductive toxicity related to the environment and the workplace is developing. With a high level of media interest, these trends will undoubtedly increase over the coming years, and we thought it important in the context of this book that health care professionals are aware of the evidence linking our environment to our reproductive wellbeing.

We hope that this book will prove to be useful to medical, pharmaceutical and nursing colleagues who are at the receiving end of enquiries from patients. More generally, we would feel encouraged if this book helped all health care professionals to be aware of the very emotive issue of sexual dysfunction provoked by drugs.

Robert Forman
Susanna Gilmour-White
Nathalie Forman

1

Sexual and reproductive function

Sperm production and transport

Male reproductive anatomy

The male reproductive tract consists of the testes, which produce sperm, and a series of ducts and tubes allowing the sperm and seminal plasma to be secreted (see Fig. 1.1). Testicular sperm drain into the epididymis which is a single convoluted tubule opening into the vas deferens. The epididymis is divided into three regions, the caput, corpus and caudum. Sperm concentration and maturative changes occur in the caput and corpus regions and are regulated by the concentrations of hormones and proteins within the epididymis. The cauda acts as a sperm reservoir where sperm may be stored for several weeks before being released into the vas deferens. The vas is approximately 25 cm long and passes into the peritoneal cavity via the inguinal canal before opening into the urethra. Secretions from the accessory glands, the seminal vesicles and prostate, drain into the urethra to form the bulk of the semen or seminal plasma. The bulbourethral glands produce a small amount of seminal fluid.

Anatomy of the testis

The testes are paired organs consisting of an outer capsule, the tunica albuginea, the seminiferous tubules, which form sperm, and the interstitial tissue (see Fig. 1.2). The seminiferous tubules, which occupy most of the volume of the testis, are contained in lobules (of which there are approximately 300), each lobule containing between one and four tubules. The tubules are composed of *germ cells* and *Sertoli cells*. The sperm produced in the seminiferous tubules pass into the ductus efferentes and rete testis before reaching the epididymis. The interstitial tissue fills the spaces between the seminiferous tubules and contains the *Leydig cells*.

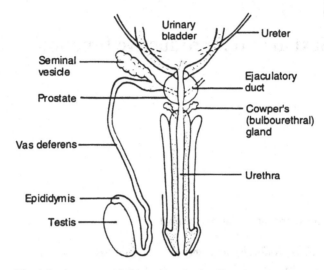

Fig. 1.1. Anatomy of the male reproductive tract.

Testicular function

Spermatogenesis

The primitive germ cells in the testis divide to form spermatogonia. These are present from fetal life and remain inactive until the prepubertal period when they start dividing by mitosis to form the pool of cells that will either proceed into spermatogenesis, form replacement germ cells or degenerate. The change from spermatogonia, which are diploid (46 chromosomes), to spermatids, which only contain the haploid number of chromosomes (23), is termed spermatogenesis. This is illustrated in Fig. 1.3. Each spermatogonium will form a primary spermatocyte that will divide into two secondary spermatocytes. These will each divide into two spermatids. The number of spermatogonia entering the cycle of spermatogenesis is under the control of follicle-stimulating hormone (FSH) and luteinising hormone (LH). However, the timing of each stage of spermatogenesis is not hormone dependent. In humans, spermatogenesis can only be completed if the testis is at a lower temperature than the rest of the body. This is achieved by the testes being outside the body core in the scrotum.

Spermiogenesis

Spermatids do not resemble mature spermatozoa. They are spherical cells with a large nucleus. The process of development into mature spermatozoa

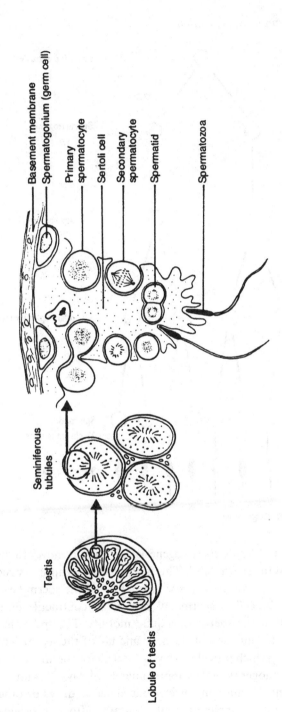

Basement membrane
Spermatogonium (germ cell)
Primary spermatocyte
Sertoli cell
Secondary spermatocyte
Spermatid
Spermatozoa
Seminiferous tubules
Testis
Lobule of testis

Fig. 1.2. Site of sperm formation within the testis.

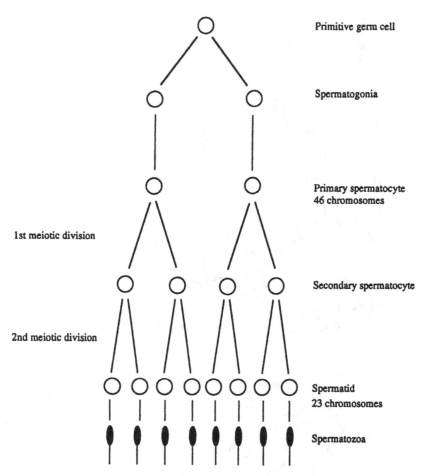

Fig. 1.3. Spermatogenesis.

is called spermiogenesis. During spermiogenesis, the nucleus moves to one side of the cell to form the sperm head. This is covered by a cap-like structure, the acrosome, which overlies approximately half of the sperm head. At the other end of the cell, a sperm tail containing contractile fibres develops. This will allow the sperm to acquire motility. The sperm mid piece develops around the junction of the head and tail of the sperm. This contains mitochondria, which provide an energy source for sperm motility.

The process of spermiogenesis takes approximately 74 days. It is important to be aware of this because any deleterious effect of drugs or other noxious agents may not be apparent until 3 months after the original insult.

Sertoli cells

The Sertoli cell is a highly complex cell with several important functions. It envelops the developing sperm cell and because of its ability to regulate its immediate environment is sometimes called a 'nurse cell'.

The functions of the Sertoli cell can be summarised as follows:

Maintenance of blood-testis barrier. The Sertoli cell and germ cells rest on the basal layer of the seminiferous epithelium. Tight junctions between adjacent Sertoli cells form the most significant part of the blood-testis barrier. The environment of developing sperm is, therefore, protected by the Sertoli cells and toxic agents in the blood are excluded. The only fluid surrounding the developing sperm is that secreted by the Sertoli cells (Fig. 1.2).

Secretion of proteins. The Sertoli cell secretes up to 100 proteins into both the seminiferous tubular fluid and the bloodstream. One of the most important is androgen-binding protein (ABP). This regulates the action of testosterone and other androgens within the male reproductive tract. Only the free unbound form of testosterone is biologically active. An increase or decrease in the amount of ABP will, therefore, influence both sperm production and sperm function.

Secretion of hormones. Sertoli cell action is influenced by FSH from the anterior pituitary. Inhibin, one of the major hormones produced by Sertoli cells, is so called because of its negative feedback on FSH secretion. This enables fine modulation of Sertoli cell action.

Leydig cells

Under the influence of pituitary LH, the Leydig cells are the main site of androgen synthesis, producing testosterone, which has to be metabolised to its biologically active form, dihydrotestosterone (DHT). Testosterone acts by negative feedback to reduce the secretion of LH from the pituitary.

Male sexual function

Many drugs affect sexual function in the male by interfering with the mechanisms responsible for erection or ejaculation. These drugs may act centrally to inhibit cerebral control or they may exert specific influence on either the blood supply or the innervation of the penis or accessory glands.

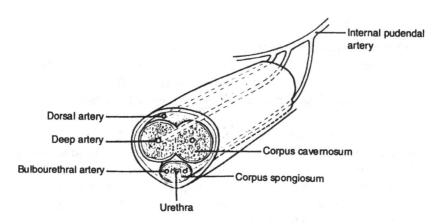

Fig. 1.4. Anatomy of the penis.

The following section discusses the physiological processes involved in normal sexual function.

Erection

Anatomy of the penis

The erectile tissue of the human penis is composed of three muscle bundles, two corpora cavernosa situated dorsally and the corpus spongiosum, which surrounds the urethra. Within each muscle bundle lie many cavernous spaces separated by trabeculae, which contain smooth muscle (see Fig. 1.4) The control of blood flow into and out of these cavernous spaces is responsible for erection and detumescence.

Vascular supply to the penis

The internal pudendal arteries provide the blood supply to the penis (see Fig. 1.4). Each internal pudendal artery gives off a bulbar branch and a urethral artery that supply the corpus spongiosum. The internal pudendal artery then divides into the deep and dorsal arteries of the penis. The deep artery runs through each corpus cavernosum, giving off helical arteries that subdivide into end arteries. These end arteries provide blood flow directly into the cavernous spaces. The dorsal artery remains external. There are many anastomotic connections between all the arteries. Venous drainage parallels the arterial blood supply.

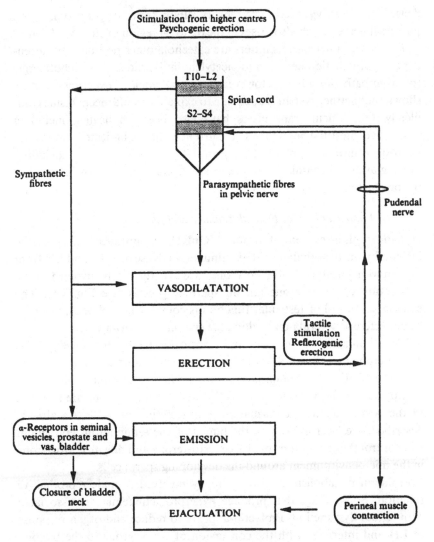

Fig. 1.5. Neurological control of male sexual function.

Innervation of the penis

The penis is innervated by both the autonomic (parasympathetic and sympathetic) and somatic systems (see Fig. 1.5). These supply the smooth muscle of the corpora as well as the blood vessels. The autonomic supply arises from the pelvic plexus, which receives both parasympathetic and sympathetic systems. The sympathetic supply originates between T10 and L2 and the parasympathetic from S2 to S4. The parasympathetic fibres condense into the pelvic nerve. The sensory supply from the penis runs in the pudendal nerve, which also arises in the S2 to S4 region of the spinal cord.

The classical neurotransmitters are catecholamines produced by adrenergic (sympathetic) nerves and acetylcholine produced by cholinergic (parasympathetic) fibres. However, pharmacological experiments have shown that neither system is adequate to explain erectile mechanisms completely. Other neurotransmitters have also been implicated, including vasoactive intestinal peptide (VIP). Current evidence indicates that several neurotransmitters previously postulated as active, including prostaglandins, histamine and amino acids, are probably not involved in the production of erection in humans.

Endocrinology of testicular and sexual function

Gonadotrophin-releasing hormone (GnRH) is produced in pulsatile fashion by the hypothalamus. This stimulates release of FSH and LH from the anterior pituitary. These hormones are synergistically involved in the production of testosterone and in spermatogenesis (see Fig. 1.6). The endocrine control of testicular function is complex but relevant, as drugs can interfere at several points along the endocrine pathway.

LH stimulates the production of testosterone by the Leydig cells. Testosterone as well as FSH from the anterior pituitary are the main hormones regulating the seminiferous epithelium. They mediate this regulation by acting on the Sertoli cell. Both FSH and testosterone are involved in the regulation of the formation and secretion of ABP. As already described, the level of ABP in the lumen of the seminiferous epithelium will control the concentration of free testosterone and dihydrotestosterone in the microenvironment around the developing sperm cells.

Prolactin metabolism is also indirectly involved in male reproductive function. Some drugs that produce hyperprolactinaemia are associated with sexual dysfunction. Prolactin appears to reduce end-organ response to LH and interferes with the conversion of testosterone to the biologically active form, dihydrotestosterone.

Drug-induced changes in FSH and LH metabolism can, therefore, affect testosterone levels, leading to sexual dysfunction and/or disorders of spermatogenesis. In the clincial setting, low testosterone levels tend to be associated with reduced libido rather than erectile dysfunction.

Vascular changes at erection

Erection is a phenomenon produced by arterial vasodilatation associated with smooth muscle relaxation of the corpora. This enables blood to flow

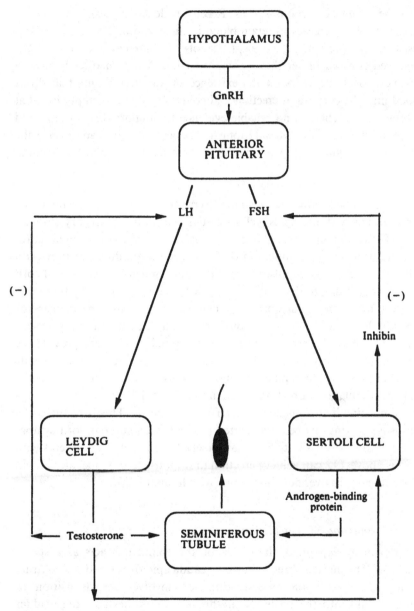

Fig. 1.6. Hormonal control of testicular function.

into the dilated cavernous spaces. Recent evidence suggests that venous resistance also increases to retain blood in the corpora. The rise in venous resistance is probably a consequence of external compression by the engorged corpora rather than vasoconstriction. Many theories have been advanced over the years on the existence of vascular shunts that divert blood into the corpora at erection and conversely open to empty blood at detumescence. There is no reliable evidence to support this concept, and simple dilatation of the arterial supply to the penis and the trabeculae of the corpora is adequate to explain the vascular mechanism involved in erection.

Neural control of erection

Erection can be produced in response to psychogenic stimuli arising in the cerebral cortex (fantasy) as well as visual and auditory sensory stimulation. These stimuli descend from the higher centres to the spinal cord. Alternatively, tactile stimulation of the penis can produce erection via a reflex arc that sends impulses through sacral segments of the spinal cord without ascending to the brain (see Fig. 1.5). The parasympathetic supply appears to be the most important neurological control mechanism for erection. Physiological information from animal experiments has provided some data, but observations in men with spinal cord injury provide the most reliable information in humans. Lesions of the sacral cord segments abolish the sacral spinal reflex arc and the penis does not respond to tactile genital stimulation. Erections may, however, still be produced by psychogenic stimuli such as erotic material and fantasy. This is mediated by pathways linking the cerebral cortex to the thoracolumbar cord sympathetic outflow from T10 to T12. Conversely, less than 10% of patients with lesions above T12 can achieve erection in response to pyschogenic stimuli. This increases to over 50% in patients with lumbar lesions.

Emission and ejaculation

As previously explained, the cauda of the epididymis acts as a sperm reservoir. The muscle fibres around the cauda epididymis and vas contract during the ejaculation process. Emission involves the deposition of seminal fluid into the posterior urethra. At the same time, the bladder neck closes to prevent retrograde passage of semen into the bladder. Contraction of the vas deferens during emission and closure of the bladder neck are under the control of sympathetic nerve fibres (see Fig. 1.5). These same fibres innervate the prostate and seminal vesicles, which produce nearly all of the seminal fluid. Factors interfering with the function of these nerve fibres can, therefore, lead to a number of complaints, including retrograde ejaculation (caused by failure of closure of the bladder neck) or aspermia (absence of semen or 'dry orgasm'.) These factors include trauma to the the pelvic nerve plexus and treatment with α-adrenergic-blocking agents, which interfere with the action of noradrenaline released from sympathetic nerve terminals.

Ejaculation is the process leading to the expulsion of semen from the posterior urethra via the urethral meatus as a consequence of contractions of the striated perineal muscles. These are innervated by the pudendal nerve, which is somatic in origin.

Reproductive function in females

Oogenesis

Primitive egg cells in the female are called oogonia. They divide rapidly during fetal life to reach a maximum number of approximately 7 million by the sixth month of pregnancy. They then remain suspended partway through the first meiotic division and remain in that state for up to 50 years. At this stage, they are known as oocytes. The first meiotic division is only finally completed at ovulation and the second meiotic division follows fertilisation. From 24 weeks of fetal life until the menopause there is a rapid loss of oocytes by atresia (degeneration). A baby is born with 2 million oocytes but by puberty only 400 000 remain. These oocytes are surrounded by a single layer of granulosa cells, and the oocyte granulosa complex at this stage is called a primordial follicle. Some follicles start development during childhood but they will all degenerate.

During reproductive life, follicles develop in waves from small primary follicles through a series of eight stages to preovulatory follicles, which will rupture and release the egg in response to the appropriate gonadotrophin stimulation. It has been estimated that the duration of time for a small primary follicle to develop into a preovulatory follicle is approximately 85 days (i.e. nearly three menstrual cycles). The entry of groups of follicles into the cycle of follicular growth is not dependent on gonadotrophins. However, when FSH levels rise at the beginning of the menstrual cycle there will be a group of follicles of a certain size containing a critical number of granulosa cells that are able to 'catch the wave' and become recruited for that particular menstrual cycle. In natural cycles, one of this developing subgroup will be selected to become dominant. The others will advance only partway along the wave and then degenerate. In this

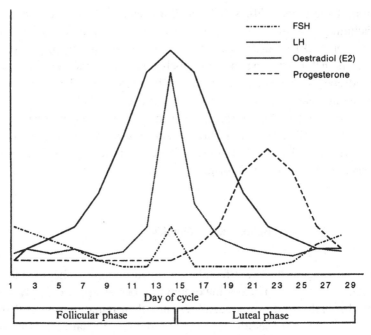

Fig. 1.7. Hormonal changes during the menstrual cycle.

way, 99.9% of the 400 000 eggs present in the human ovary at the onset of reproductive life will degenerate and only an average of 360 eggs will be ovulated and stand a chance of being fertilised to commence a new human life.

Hormonal control of ovulation

Hormonal changes during a typical menstrual cycle are illustrated in Fig. 1.7. Each month, FSH levels begin to rise just before the onset of menstruation in the late luteal phase. FSH stimulates the granulosa cells of follicles between 1 and 5 mm in diameter to produce oestradiol (E2). As the oestradiol level rises in the second half of the follicular phase it exerts a negative feedback effect on the pituitary gland production of FSH. Only the follicle destined to ovulate (dominant follicle) is able to retain the reduced level of FSH selectively and continue to produce oestradiol. This is probably because it has the most abundant blood supply. The other follicles that had been recruited start to degenerate. Once oestradiol production from the dominant follicle reaches a critical level, it triggers a surge in LH production from the pituitary by positive feedback.

The LH surge induces a number of significant alterations to the follicle.

Resumption of first meiotic division. As described previously, the oocyte has been in a state of suspended animation (arrested halfway through the first meiotic division) since embryonic life. During this arrested stage, it contained the diploid number of chromosomes packed into the nucleus (germinal vesicle). The LH surge induces the resumption of the first meiotic division. The chromosome number is divided into two equal halves, with one portion remaining within the egg cytoplasm (which now becomes haploid) and the second portion being expelled as the first polar body. At the completion of this division, meiosis then arrests again. The second meiotic division only occurs if fertilisation of the egg by the sperm takes place. Otherwise the ovulated egg degenerates.

Luteinisation of granulosa cells. Protein synthesis induced by the LH surge causes a change in the secretory product of granulosa cells from oestradiol to progesterone. Progesterone influences the endometrium making it receptive to embryo implantation should a fertilised egg arrive in the uterine cavity.

Follicular rupture. LH induces an increase in follicular blood flow, which leads to a rise in follicular volume but no change in intrafollicular pressure. There is rapid development of oedema and increased vascular permeability of the follicular wall. This is accompanied by the release of prostaglandins, histamines and noradrenaline. The net effect of these changes is the release of plasmin, which breaks down the collagen in the follicular wall leading to rupture of the follicle and release of the oocyte.

Female sexual function

The female sexual response was defined by the classic studies of Masters and Johnson, who described four phases: excitement, plateau, orgasm and resolution. The excitement phase is accompanied by increased blood flow to the pelvic organs secondary to vascular dilatation. This causes increased vaginal lubrication. Adequate lubrication only occurs if circulating oestradiol levels are normal. Other changes in the excitement phase include clitoral engorgement and relaxation of the vaginal muscles.

Should sexual stimulation continue, the woman enters the plateau phase in which the outer third of the vagina becomes engorged with blood, and this stage may pass on to orgasm. Orgasm consists of involuntary rhythmic contractions of vaginal and pelvic muscles associated with an intense

pleasurable sensation. Finally, during the relaxation phase the above physiological changes resolve.

The neural mechanisms controlling the different phases of sexual
response in females are unclear. However, it is apparent that both central
and autonomic nervous systems are implicated.

Disorders of female sexual function

Female sexual dysfunction has been less investigated than the male coun-
terpart, although it appears to be at least as common as in men. Very little
is known about the adverse effects of drugs on female sexual function, as
women involved in studies have not generally been questioned about
sexual side effects.

Some rational mechanisms can be deduced for sexual side effects caused
by certain types of drug. The assumption underlying these is that the
physiological control of male and female sexual responses is analagous,
although there are few data to substantiate these assumptions.
Vasodilatation and vaginal lubrication in the female, therefore, are probably equivalent to erection in the male. The central and peripheral neu-
rovascular control of orgasm should be the same in both sexes.

2

Antihypertensive therapy

Hypertension is one of the most frequent reasons for medical consultations in the developed world. In the USA alone, 35 million people are affected and 2 million die from hypertension and hypertensive-related illnesses each year. Hypertension is frequently asymptomatic and is usually detected only by screening.

Compliance with antihypertensive medication

Difficulty can be experienced in persuading patients of the need for drug therapy particularly as they are often asymptomatic. Compliance with therapy is frequently poor especially when side effects occur. Trials performed to assess this show that between 8 and 35% of all treated patients discontinue therapy because of adverse effects. Although a few patients withdraw for serious side effects, such as bradycardia, the majority stop treatment for symptoms interfering with the quality of life. Patients may willingly report socially acceptable side effects such as nausea, lethargy or headaches, but there is increasing evidence that they may not volunteer information about sexual dysfunction. It has been known for many years that certain drugs may provoke sexual dysfunction, but many medical practitioners are unaware of the number of therapeutic classes of antihypertensive drug that have been reported to modify sexual function and behaviour. It is also important during the monitoring of antihypertensive therapy that prescribers directly question men and women on whether they are experiencing sexual problems.

Gender differences

There is certainly a gender difference in reports of sexual dysfunction related to antihypertensive therapy. For example, in the Hypertension

Detection and Follow-up Programme in the USA, 8.3% of men but only 0.4% of women stopped their antihypertensive drug because of sexual side effects (Curb *et al.*, 1985). A recent report on hypertension in women from the Working Group on Womens' Health of the Society of General Internal Medicine quite rightly concludes that the reported low incidence of sexual dysfunction in women on hypertensive therapy is because the appropriate questions have not been posed (Anastos *et al.*, 1991). This is probably a consequence of study design. Many studies rely on patients volunteered complaints, a method that is known to be associated with significant underreporting. Others are structured so that there is no possibility of a response from a female subject: For example, 'have you experienced any difficulty with erection or ejaculation?' As the authors of the above report state, ' Penile erection in men is physiologically analogous to lubrication and clitoral engorgement in women: male ejaculation is analogous to female orgasm. It is, therefore, reasonable to suppose that medications that cause sexual dysfunction in men may do so in women as well'.

Effect of hypertension on sexual function

Untreated hypertensive patients are more troubled by sexual disorders than non-hypertensive subjects. A group of 163 untreated hypertensive men who were enrolled in a trial of antihypertensive medication were questioned on their sexual symptoms. Of these, 33% complained of decreased libido, 22% problems with gaining an erection, 23% problems with maintaining an erection and 17% a disturbance of ejaculation (Croog *et al.*, 1988). Another study showed that 25% of treated hypertensives complained of impotence compared with 17% of untreated hypertensives and 7% of normotensive controls (Bulpitt, Dollery & Carne, 1976). This figure for controls is thought to represent accurately the incidence of impotence in the general population. The incidence is increased in diabetic hypertensive patients because of diabetic peripheral autonomic neuropathy and microvascular arteriolar damage. Other factors such as age, smoking and alcohol consumption are also relevant. These are often ignored in clinical trials but independently correlate with sexual function. Therefore, some caution is needed before automatically assuming a causal relationship between an individual antihypertensive agent and sexual dysfunction.

Choice of antihypertensive drug

Until recently, hypertension was treated initially using either a thiazide diuretic or a β-blocker. If the response was poor, both therapies were administered concurrently. If the combination was still ineffective a centrally acting agent, such as methyldopa, or a peripheral vasodilator was added to the regimen. The disadvantage of this approach is the cumulative adverse effects of the different drugs and the poor compliance often seen when drug combinations are administered.

Recent pharmacological developments have led to a range of single-agent therapies now being available for the first-line treatment of hypertension. The most important recent trend appears to be a move away from highly regimented treatment protocols to individualisation of therapy. As concurrent medical disorders are present in over 50% of hypertensive patients, this can be reflected in prescribing patterns. For example, patients with angina are more likely to receive a β-blocker or calcium-channel blocker, those with diabetes mellitus or hyperlipidaemia are more likely to receive a calcium-channel blocker or angiotensin converting enzyme (ACE) inhibitor, etc. Although single-agent therapy is beneficial for patients' compliance, long-term safety and efficacy data on these more recently marketed products are less extensive than for diuretics and β-blockers. Based on the data that are available, minor side effects may be more common but as seen below the incidence of sexual dysfunction may be reduced.

Centrally acting drugs

Methyldopa

The antihypertensive effect of methyldopa is related to its metabolism to α-methyl-noradrenaline. This stimulates central inhibitory (sympathetic) α_2-adrenergic receptors, acts as a false transmitter and also reduces renin activity. Methyldopa has many well-documented detrimental effects on sexual function. In men, these include the inability to maintain erection (20–80%), ejaculatory disturbances (7–19%), decreased libido (7–14%) and gynaecomastia. These have been reported at standard therapeutic doses (Buffum, 1982). In women, decreased libido, painful breast enlargement and delayed or absent orgasm have been described. There have been isolated reports in women of amenorrhoea and galactorrhoea.

The reported incidence of impotence is high, although study design is very relevant. For example, an interview-based study of 30 men revealed an 80% incidence in patients taking 1–2 g per day of methyldopa. A much larger placebo-controlled single-blind study demonstrated impotence in only 20%. This was the same as in a group of untreated hypertensive men. In another study, impairment of libido has been described in 15% and impairment of ejaculation was self reported by 7% of treated men. However 53% of this same group of patients complained of ejaculatory disturbance following detailed questioning. In general, studies in which patients volunteered symptoms reported a lower incidence of side effects than when specific questions on sexual dysfunction were asked (Smith and Talbert, 1986).

The sexual dysfunction associated with methyldopa may be related to one of several mechanisms. It inhibits sympathetic outflow from the brain-stem, which directly influences erection. As a false transmitter, it reduces noradrenergic stimulation of postsynaptic α-adrenoceptors, which can affect ejaculation. The decrease in libido can be explained by depletion of central neurotransmitters as well as by the sedative and depressant proper-ties of the drug. Depression may also be a factor in erectile dysfunction. Methyldopa induces hyperprolactinaemia, which explains the reported amenorrhoea and galactorrhoea. Additionally, it has been suggested that high prolactin decreases pulsatile gonadotrophin-releasing hormone secre-tion, leading to a reduction in serum testosterone levels. This may also be related to impotence and reduction of libido.

Clonidine

The mode of action of clonidine is similar to that of methyldopa and it is, therefore, not altogether surprising that erectile failure and reduced libido have been associated with its use. As with methyldopa, the incidence of these complications varies greatly between studies. Impotence occurs in 4–70% of patients and reduced libido was common in one small study (Buffum, 1982). A few cases of retrograde ejaculation have been reported (McWaine & Procci, 1988).

Vasodilators

Hydralazine

Hydralazine is a peripherally acting vasodilator that relaxes vascular smooth muscle. There are very few reports of undesired effects on sexual function and most of these implicate combination therapy such as hydralazine and propranolol or hydralazine and a thiazide diuretic. There has been one report of priapism developing during hydralazine therapy and the suggestion has been made that the drug even has aphrodisiac properties. However, this occurred in a patient who was changed from a thiazide diuretic (known to cause decreased libido) to hydralazine (Stevenson & Umstead, 1984).

Diuretics

Thiazides

Thiazides act by producing a reduction in blood volume associated with initial diuresis. Thereafter, a sustained vasodilator action is probably responsible for their effects. A Medical Research Council Working Party in 1981 reported a 16% incidence of impotence in patients taking thiazide diuretics after 12 weeks of treatment (Medical Research Council Working Party, 1981). A recent randomised study of diuretics in mild hypertension showed a significant increase in sexual dysfunction compared with placebo. This was still observable after controlling for confounding factors such as older age, diabetes mellitus and use of other (non-diuretic) antihypertensive therapy. The disorders noted included a reduction in libido, difficulty in obtaining or maintaining erection and problems with ejaculation. Patients on diuretics were two to six times more likely to experience sexual dysfunction than those on placebo (Chang *et al.*, 1991). Reduced vaginal lubrication has been described in females. A recent large multicentre study evaluated the effects of a thiazide diuretic (chlorthalidone), atenolol and different diets on sexual function. In a group of men on their normal diet receiving chlorthalidone, 28% experienced problems with erection compared with 3% of those on placebo and a normal diet. However, men on chlorthalidone with a weight-reducing diet were less affected. In this study, the authors specifically questioned women about sexual side effects. In the group of women treated with chlorthalidone, 22% of those on a normal diet but only 8% of those on a weight-reducing diet had a worsening of their sexual problems. This illustrates the multifactorial influences on sexual function in hypertensive individuals (Wassertheil-Smoller *et al.*, 1991).

A recent study of men starting antihypertensive medication for the first time demonstrated a significant increase in anorgasmia within 30 days of commencing medication in men receiving hydrochlorthiazide (Kroner, Mulligan & Briggs, 1993).

The mechanisms behind the sexual side effects are not readily apparent as thiazides lack significant hormonal, autonomic or central nervous system effects. Decreased peripheral resistance has been suggested, but sexual side effects have not been reported with vasodilators that have a similar mode of action. It has also been proposed that it may be the result of a direct effect of thiazides on smooth muscle or by interference with catecholamine responsiveness.

Spironolactone

This potassium-sparing diuretic has been associated with a variety of sexual side effects. Dose-dependent gynaecomastia is well recognised and occurred in 100% of patients treated with 400 mg/day (used to differentiate primary from secondary hyperaldosteronism); 30% also developed impotence. Both recovered following discontinuation of spironolactone (Spark & Melby, 1968). Similar effects have been less commonly reported on lower doses of 50–100 mg/day (Buffum, 1982; Smith and Talbert, 1986). The 400 mg study also included women all of whom developed menstrual irregularities.

Spironolactone is an antiandrogen (it is also used in the treatment of hirsutism) and the adverse sexual effects are probably hormonally induced. It prevents the binding of dihydrotestosterone to androgen receptors, which leads to increased metabolic clearance of testosterone and increased peripheral conversion to oestradiol. In women, the menstrual irregularity is probably related to defective ovulation and could be a cause of subfertility. High doses of spironolactone inhibit 17-hydroxylase, which is an important component of the steroid biosynthetic pathway. 17-Hydroxylase blockade causes anovulation in women.

Adrenergic neurone blockers

Reserpine

This drug is not currently in frequent use, but it has been implicated in causing decreased libido in nearly 50% of patients. Impotence and ejaculatory failure are less common, with quoted incidences of 33% and 14%, respectively. Decreased libido has also been described in women on reserpine therapy. These side effects may be mediated by catecholamine depletion, which would affect erection, ejaculation and sexual desire. Possibly depression, induced by reserpine, is also a factor.

Guanethidine

Guanethidine has potent effects on sexual physiology. It is a postganglionic adrenergic neurone blocker and acts peripherally to prevent noradrenaline uptake into intraneuronal storage granules. It also probably inhibits the release of catecholamines by nerve stimuli. Guanethidine suppresses responses mediated by both α- and β-adrenoceptors.

The main problems induced by guanethidine involve ejaculatory mechanisms. This may be because the drug seems to exert its greatest effect on postganglionic α_1-adrenoceptors in the vas deferens. Failure of ejaculation may be caused by either failure of emission ('dry' orgasm) or retrograde ejaculation. The incidence varies from 4 to 100%, depending on the study, and occurs in doses in excess of 25 mg/day (Buffum, 1982). In one large study of hypertensive men receiving guanethidine and a diuretic, 66% of patients reported ejaculatory disturbance but this was only described by 14% of patients taking a diuretic alone. Retrograde ejaculation occurs because guanethidine impairs sympathetically mediated closure of the internal urethral sphincter while leaving the reflex arc portion of ejaculation intact. Erectile disturbances have been reported to occur in many patients on guanethidine possibly because of shunting of blood away from the penis. However, guanethidine does not inhibit parasympathetic function so the mechanism by which this occurs is not clear. Furthermore, several reports have described reduced libido with this drug and this has been ascribed to a centrally active sympatholytic mechanism. However, because of its polar structure, it is unlikely that guanethidine crosses the blood-brain barrier in sufficient concentrations to exert this effect. It has been proposed that the impotence and decreased libido may be secondary to depression caused by ejaculatory difficulties. Also in many of these studies, other drugs have been concomitantly administered.

Guanethidine is now used less frequently in managing hypertensive patients, in part because of its high incidence of side effects, including sexual disturbances. These effects seem to be dose related and are completely reversible on discontinuing the drug.

Bethanidine and *debrisoquine* are both adrenergic neurone blockers with similar side effect profiles to guanethidine.

Alpha-blockers

Phenoxybenzamine

This is an α-adrenergic blocker that impedes the action of noradrenaline at the neuroeffector junction. It also inhibits the reuptake of catecholamines. The main sexual effects are related to ejaculation. Both failure of emission and retrograde ejaculation have been described, although this latter phenomenon has only been suggested in one report, which described the passage of white urine following orgasm. The incidence of ejaculation disorders varies widely between 4.5 and 100%. Problems have been noted at doses of 5–70 mg/day (Buffum, 1982; 1992). The incidence of side effects are highest with high doses. It is likely that the effects on ejaculation are related to inhibition of α-adrenoceptors in the prostate, seminal vesicles and epididymis, which are involved in the production and transport of seminal fluid. Disorders of ejaculation also occur with *indoramin,* which has a similar mechanism of action to phenoxybenzamine.

Prazosin

Prazosin is another α-adrenergic blocker acting by competitive antagonism at the postsynaptic α_1-adrenoceptor. Failure of ejaculation has been reported but is rare compared with that seen with phenoxybenzamine (only 0.6 to 4%). Unspecified sexual disorders occurred in 9% of patients in one study. This can occur at doses between 3 and 20 mg/day (Buffum, 1982). In a review of over 900 men on prazosin, impotence was only recorded in 0.6% (Smith & Talbert, 1986). In one study, 19 diabetic hypertensive individuals with sexual dysfunction taking clonidine or methyldopa were changed to prazosin; 79% had normal or improved sexual function after 2 months. To rule out a placebo effect, this was later shown to correlate with objective measurements of nocturnal penile tumescence (Lipson, 1984).

Priapism has also been described in several reports, occurring one to three months after starting therapy and resolving when prazosin was discontinued. Presumably this is secondary to α blockade-induced vasodilatation, leading to increased blood flow to the corpora cavernosum. Several of the reports of prazosin-induced priapism have been in patients with renal failure. It has been suggested that the hypoproteinaemia accompanying uraemia may result in an decrease in the fraction of drug bound to plasma proteins, thereby increasing the active free fraction and potentiating the effect. However, prazosin has been recommended as a good second-line antihypertensive in sexually active individuals.

Beta-blockers

Propranolol

Beta-blockers have complex mechanisms of action. They reduce cardiac output, alter baroreceptor sensitivity and block peripheral β-adrenoceptors. Some β-blockers including propranolol, also reduce renin activity. Propranolol is a non-specific β_1- and β_2-receptor-blocking agent. Certain β-blockers, notably propranolol, metoprolol and oxprenolol, are lipid soluble. The consequence of this is that these drugs can cross the blood–brain barrier to exert a central nervous system effect.

Impotence appears to be the major adverse influence of propranolol on sexual function. A Medical Research Council Working Party reported impotence in 14% of propranolol-treated patients after therapy for three months compared with 9% in controls (Medical Research Council Working Party, 1981). This difference is not convincing. However, the effects may be dose related and are more frequent in doses greater than 120 mg/day. In a review of the sexual side effects of propranolol, Smith and Talbert (1986) found impotence in 5 to 15% of patients.

Patients being treated with higher doses may have more severe underlying disease and propranolol has been used to treat angina as well as hypertension in some of the studies using higher dosages. This introduces an additional variable. It has been suggested that erectile failure and dysfunction is caused by β blockade, which leads to unopposed α-adrenoceptor-mediated vasoconstriction and affects blood flow to the corpora cavernosa. However, a central action related to lipid solubility cannot be excluded. In one case, erectile dysfunction secondary to propranolol was relieved when atenolol (a less lipophilic agent) was substituted (Bathen, 1978). Decreased libido has been described in 1–4% of both men and women taking propranolol and is probably related to central effects (Smith and Talbert, 1986). Case reports have appeared describing both failure of ejaculation and Peyronie's disease in patients taking propranolol.

It has been suggested that lipid-soluble agents including propranolol can adsorb onto the sperm membrane. *In vitro* in high concentrations propranolol can reduce sperm motility directly through a local anaesthetic effect on the sperm membrane. In the clinical situation, this is probably not of any consequence, as therapeutic doses are about 1000 times lower than the dose required to immobilise sperm.

Atenolol

Atenolol is a specific β_1-adrenoceptor blocker. Sexual side effects are very uncommon, presumably because the drug is cardiospecific with no effect on skin or resting muscle blood flow. A study of 543 men on atenolol reported an incidence of impotence of only 0.2% (Heel *et al.*, 1979). However, the same study only reported that 0.5% of men on propranolol experienced impotence. As described previously, propranolol-induced impotence has been reversed by changing therapy to atenolol.

Metoprolol

The same considerations apply to metoprolol as atenolol, as this drug is also cardiospecific. Isolated reports of disturbances of libido and potency are mentioned in the data sheet supplied by the manufacturers. There were no reports of sexual problems in one study of over 10 000 hypertensive patients treated with metoprolol (Buffum, 1982). Atenolol and, to a lesser extent, metoprolol have reduced lipid solubility compared with propranolol. This will reduce the possibility of central nervous system effects.

Timolol

Several reports have described impotence in patients treated with intraocular timolol for glaucoma that resolved on withdrawing the therapy. Timolol is a non-specific β-blocker so these findings are not unexpected. A recent review identifies 18 reported instances of impotence, nine of decreased libido and one of reduced ejaculate volume when timolol was administered by the intraocular route (Buffum, 1992). No data are currently available for oral therapy, but impotence is described in the data sheet.

Combined α- and β-blockers

Labetalol

Labetalol blocks α_1-, β_1- and β_2-adrenoceptors. The side effect profile can be related to its mechanism of action. Blockade of α_1-adrenoceptors causes delayed ejaculation, delayed detumescence and priapism. In one study, laboratory investigations were performed in six volunteers on doses of 100 and 300 mg labetalol. Labetalol delayed ejaculation in a dose-dependent manner and delayed detumescence measured objectively using plethysmography. In this study, there was no effect on either the attainment or maintenance of erection (Buffum, 1992).

Ejaculation failure has also been reported clinically. There has been one report of priapism with the drug, but this occurred in an individual undergoing haemodialysis, which is also known to be associated with priapism (Law *et al.*, 1980).

One study in healthy women has demonstrated reduced vaginal lubrication in women taking labetalol compared with those taking propranol and placebo (Riley & Riley, 1981).

Tyrosine hydroxylase inhibitors

Metirosine

Metirosine is mainly used in patients with phaeochromocytoma and is not recommended for use in essential hypertension. The manufacturer's data sheet lists impotence and failure of ejaculation as possible side effects, but this may be related to the sedative effects of this drug.

Calcium-channel blockers

Calcium antagonists such as *nifedipine* and *verapamil* decrease coronary and vascular smooth muscle tone by blocking calcium influx into cells. There are few clinical reports of this class of drug being associated with sexual dysfunction. A report described three cases of impotence in 14 patients treated for arrhythmias and angina with verapamil and digoxin. In two patients, symptoms developed within 4 weeks. In the remaining patient, impotence only occurred 8 months later (King *et al.*, 1983). Another report describes a 45-year-old man admitted to hospital with suicidal depression and impotence 4 months after starting verapamil for hypertension. Within 36 hours of stopping therapy, he experienced four erections and the depression had resolved (Fogelman, 1988). One placebo-controlled study suggested a decrease in erectile firmness in older men on nifedipine (Morrissette *et al.*, 1993).

The mechanism of impotence is unclear. Calcium-channel blockade might be expected to relax smooth muscle, which would increase vascular engorgement of the penis and hence potentiate erection. It has been suggested that impotence may in some way be a consequence of inhibition of parasympathetic nerve function, but there is little evidence to support this.

There has been recent interest in the influence of calcium-channel blockers on sperm function, following the report of failed fertilisation of eggs at *in vitro* fertilisation. The man, who was taking nifedipine for hypertension, had apparently completely normal sperm parameters but no sperm were able to bind to the 15 eggs. The authors performed further studies by comparing three groups of men, fertile sperm donors, men taking calcium-channel blockers and men who had taken calcium-channel blockers but who were switched to alternative hypotensive agents at least 3 months previously. The sperm of men taking nifedipine did not undergo a spontaneous acrosome reaction, which is an essential prerequisite for fertilisation. In the other two groups, the rate of spontaneous acrosome reaction, was normal. The acrosome reaction depends on calcium ion influx into the sperm. The authors suggested that men taking calcium-channel blockers should be switched to alternative medication prior to commencing fertility treatment (Benoff *et al.*, 1994). Another recently published *in vitro* study showed that verapamil was associated with sperm damage to the head and tail regions of the sperm, associated with reduced motility (Anand, Kanwar & Sanyal, 1994). The authors even thought that the drug could have potential as a male contraceptive!

Based on this evidence, it would appear a wise precaution to avoid calcium-channel blockers in men where the couple are trying to conceive.

Angiotensin-converting enzyme inhibitors

Captopril

ACE inhibitors promote vasodilatation by inhibiting the formation of angiotensin 2. As there is no specific effect on the autonomic nervous system, a low incidence of sexual side effects is to be expected. There are no reports indicating sexual dysfunction with captopril alone. In a study comparing the effect of captopril, propranolol and methyldopa on patients' distress over their sexual symptoms, those on captopril reported the least change from pretreatment symptoms (Croog *et al.*, 1986). Although 19% complained of worsening symptoms, the same percentage reported an improvement. Another large study looked at 30 000 patients (53% women) and noted improvements in sexual function in patients of both sexes when captopril was substituted for other antihypertensive medication (Schoenberger *et al.*, 1990). In one multicentre study of 900 men with mild hypertension, the incidence of difficulty in obtaining and maintaining erections was the same in men taking the ACE inhibitor *enalapril* as in those taking placebo (Mason, 1991). Benoff *et al.* (1994) recommend using ACE inhibitors rather than calcium-channel blockers for men in whom fertility may be a problem.

References

Anand, R. J., Kanwar, U. & Sanyal, S. N. (1994). Calcium channel antagonist verapamil modulates human spermatozoal functions. *Research in Experimental Medicine*, 194, 165–78.

Anastos, K., Charney, P., Charon, R. A., Cohen, E., Jones, C. Y., Marte, C., Swiderski, D. M., Wheat, M. E. & Williams, S. (1991). Hypertension in women: what is really known. *Annals of Internal Medicine*, 115, 287–93.

Bathen, J. (1978). Propranolol erectile dysfunction relieved. *Annals of Internal Medicine*, 88, 716–17.

Benoff, S., Cooper, G. W., Hurley, I., Mandel, F. S., Rosenfeld, D. L., Scholl, G. M., Gilbert, B. R. & Hershlag, A. (1994). The effect of calcium ion channel blockers on sperm fertilisation potential. *Fertility and Sterility*, 62, 606–17.

Buffum, J. (1982). Pharmacosexology: the effects of drugs on sexual function – a review. *Journal of Psychoactive Drugs*, 14, 5–44.

Buffum, J. (1992). Prescription drugs and sexual function. *Psychiatric Medicine*, 10, 181–98.

Bulpitt, C. J., Dollery, C. T. & Carne, S. (1976). Change in the symptoms of hypertensive patients after referral to a hospital clinic. *British Heart Journal*, 38, 121–8.

Chang, S. W., Fine, R., Siegel, D., Chesney, M., Black, D. & Hulley, S. B. (1991). The impact of diuretic therapy on reported sexual function. *Archives of Internal Medicine*, 151, 2402–8.

Croog, S. H., Levine, S., Sudilovsky, A., Baume, R. M. & Clive, J. (1988). Sexual symptoms in hypertensive patients: a clinical trial of antihypertensive medication. *Archives of Internal Medicine*, 148, 788–94.

Croog, S. H., Levine, S., Testa, M. A., Brown, B., Bulpitt, C. J., Jenkins, C. D., Klerman, G. L. & Williams, G. H. (1986). The effects of antihypertensive therapy on quality of life. *New England Journal of Medicine*, 314, 1657–64.

Curb, J. D., Borhani, N. O., Blaszkowski, T. P., Zimbaldi, N., Fotiu, S. & Williams, W. (1985). Long-term surveillance for adverse effects of antihypertensive drugs. *Journal of the American Medical Association*, 253, 3263–8.

Fogelman, J. (1988). Verapamil caused depression, confusion, and impotence. *American Journal of Psychiatry*, 145, 380.

Heel, R., Brogden, R., Speight, T. & Avery, G. (1979). Atenolol: a review of its pharmacological and therapeutic efficacy in angina pectoris and hypertension. *Drugs*, 17, 425–60.

King, B. D., Pitchon, R., Stern, E. H., Schweitzer, P., Schneider, R. R. & Weiner, I. (1983). Impotence during therapy with verapamil. *Archives of Internal Medicine*, 143, 1248–9.

Kroner, B. A., Mulligan, T. & Briggs, G. C. (1993). Effect of frequently prescribed cardiovascular medications on sexual function: a pilot study. *Annals of Pharmacotherapy*, 27, 1329–32.

Law, M. R., Copland, R. F., Armistead, J. G. & Gabriel, R. (1980). Labetalol and priapism. *British Medical Journal*, 280, 115.

Lipson, L. G. (1984). Special problems in treatment of hypertension in the patient with diabetes mellitus. *Archives of Internal Medicine*, 144, 1829–31.

Mason, I. (1991). Antihypertensives and sexual function. *Prescriber, 19 Sept*, 69–70.

McWaine, D. E. & Procci, W. R. (1988). Drug induced sexual dysfunction. *Medical Toxicology*, 3, 289–306.

Medical Research Council Working Party (1981). Adverse reactions to bendrofluazide and propranolol for the treatment of mild hypertension. *Lancet*, ii, 539–43.

Morrissette, D. L., Skinner, M. H., Hoffman, B. B., Levine, R. E. & Davidson, J. M. (1993). Effects of antihypertensive drugs atenolol and nifedipine on sexual function in older men: a placebo-controlled, crossover study. *Archives of Sexual Behaviour*, 22, 99–109.

Riley, A. J. & Riley, E. J. (1981). The effect of labetalol and propranolol on the pressor response to sexual arousal in women. *British Journal of Clinical Pharmacology*, 12, 341–4.

Schoenberger, J. A., Testa, M., Ross, A. D., Brennan, W. K. & Bannon, J. A. (1990). Efficacy, safety, and quality-of life assessment of captopril antihypertensive therapy in clinical practice. *Archives of Internal Medicine*, 150, 301–6.

Smith, P. J. & Talbert, R. L. (1986). Sexual dysfunction with antihypertensives and antipsychotic agents. *Clinical Pharmacy*, 5, 373–84.

Spark, R. F. & Melby, J. C. (1968). Aldosteronism in hypertension. *Annals of Internal Medicine*, 69, 685–91.

Stevenson, J. G. & Umstead, G. S. (1984). Sexual dysfunction due to antihypertensive agents. *Drug Intelligence and Clinical Pharmacology*, 18, 113–21.

Wassertheil-Smoller, S., Blaufox, D., Oberman, A., Davis, B. R., Swencionis, C., Knerr, M. O'C. Hawkins, C. M. & Langford, H. G. (1991). Effect of antihypertensives on sexual function and quality of life: the TAIM study. *Annals of Internal Medicine*, 114, 613–20.

3

Psychotropic and central nervous system drugs

Effect of psychiatric disease on sexual function

The relationship between psychotropic medication and sexual dysfunction is complicated by the fact that abnormalities of sexual function are common symptoms of underlying psychiatric illness. For example, impotence in untreated psychiatric patients is estimated to be as high as 70% depending on the diagnosis. In a controlled study of schizophrenic males versus healthy men, significant differences were found in most aspects of human sexuality between the groups. The failure of many studies and reports to include information regarding baseline sexual function makes interpretation of published data difficult. In some situations, the untreated patient cannot be relied upon to give an accurate sexual history even if questioned directly.

Despite these reservations, many data have accumulated, mainly from case reports but also from a handful of controlled trials, to suggest that some psychotropic medication does have a negative effect on sexual function. This may be a significant cause of non-compliance leading to psychiatric relapse.

Antipsychotics (neuroleptics)

Antipsychotic medication is often associated with sexual dysfunction, occurring in over 50% of patients in some studies (Buffum, 1982). The most common form of sexual dysfunction, seen both in male and female patients treated with neuroleptics, is decreased libido. Erectile and ejaculatory dysfunction are also common. Disturbances of orgasmic function occur less commonly. Neuroleptics have been reported to produce abnormalities in sperm morphology compared with the sperm of non-medicated schizophrenics (Nestoros, Lehmann & Ban, 1981).

Priapism has also been described in patients treated with antipsychotic medication. The mechanisms of drug-induced dysfunction with neuroleptics are complicated and may be mediated by hormonal and by both central and peripheral neurological mechanisms.

Effects on hormones

Neuroleptics commonly produce hyperprolactinaemia secondary to dopaminergic blockade. This may result in decreased libido and impotence in men. Neuroleptics may also decrease serum testosterone, resulting in diminished levels of sexual interest. Not all neuroleptics interact with testosterone and it is unclear whether neuroleptic-induced testosterone suppression occurs at central or gonadal level.

Effects on neurotransmitters

Neuroleptics interact with neurotransmitters involved in the regulation of sexual function (Pollack, Reiter & Hammerness, 1992).

Effects on dopamine. Agents that block central dopaminergic transmission decrease or suppress spontaneous sexual behaviour in rats. Neuroleptics may inhibit sexual function via this mechanism.

Effects on serotonin. Central serotonin activity may inhibit sexual behaviour. There is suggestive evidence that neuroleptics facilitate serotonergic function.

Effects on acetylcholine. Anticholinergic properties of neuroleptics may decrease sexual behaviour.

Effect on peripheral nerves

Most neuroleptics are α-adrenergic-blocking agents. This effect interferes with erection and emission/ejaculation. They have also been shown to block calcium channels, which may interfere with muscle contraction of the vas deferens (Pollack *et al.*, 1992).

Phenothiazines

Thioridazine

This neuroleptic used in the treatment of schizophrenia is well known for its sexual side effects at doses as low as 30 mg/day. In men, thioridazine was first reported to interfere with ejaculation in 1961. Since then numerous case reports and a few studies describe decreased libido, difficulty achieving and maintaining erections and inability to achieve orgasm. The drug has even been used therapeutically in an attempt to treat hypersexuality and premature ejaculation (Mitchell and Popkin, 1982).

Kotin and colleagues performed a large study investigating thioridazine-induced sexual dysfunction in sexually active schizophrenics (Kotin *et al.*, 1976). Thioridazine produced some form of sexual dysfunction in 60% of patients; 44% of thioridazine-treated patients developed difficulties achieving erection compared with 19% in patients treated with other major tranquilisers. In addition, 35% of thioridazine patients had difficulty in maintaining erection (controls 11%). Half of the thioridazine group noted changes in ejaculation, whilst this was not noted in any controls. The majority of the 28 patients with altered ejaculation had no ejaculate at orgasm, the remainder reported reduced ejaculate volume. No tests were performed to see if these men had retrograde ejaculation, but this phenomenon has been previously suggested in thioridazine-treated patients. Only one report, however, has given even indirect evidence for retrograde ejaculation; a single patient complained of passing 'white urine' following orgasm without ejaculation (Shader, 1964). Two men in the series described by Kotin and co-workers (1976) also reported pain on orgasm and one of the authors who voluntarily took a test dose of the drug and masturbated 4 hours later described a tearing suprapubic pain at orgasm, but no ejaculate was produced.

Several cases of priapism have also been described. This is thought to be related to α-adrenergic blockade.

One study showed that serum levels of testosterone and LH are lower in patients on thioridazine than in controls (Brown, Laughren & Williams, 1981).

In women, thioridazine has been reported to be associated with orgasmic dysfunction (Shen & Park, 1982; Kotin *et al.*,1976). An early study reported that amenorrhoea occurred in up to 50% of patients, but this effect is reversible and normal menstruation returned after discontinuation of thioridazine (Sandison, Whitelaw & Currie, 1960). The datasheet also mentions hyperprolactinaemia resulting in galactorrhoea, oligomenorrhoea and amenorrhoea.

Chlorpromazine

Chlorpromazine is a widely used neuroleptic. Clinically, there is little evidence of sexual dysfunction with chlorpromazine. At 125 mg/day, chlorpromazine has no more sexual side-effects than placebo. However, a case of ejaculatory failure has been reported at 1200 mg/day, as well as decreased libido and decreased erectile ability. Libido, erection and orgasm returned at 400 mg/day (Buffum, 1982).

Several cases of priapism have been reported at doses of 100 mg/day and above (Buffum, 1986). In one unusual case, priapism developed after a patient inserted a crushed chlorpromazine tablet into the urethral meatus of his penis (Jackson & Walker, 1991). One man developed priapism 5 days after a single 200 mg intramuscular dose. (Chen and Lee, 1990). Priapism is usually thought to be caused by α-adrenergic blockade but the authors of this case report argued that it may also represent a hypersensitivity reaction. Other mechanisms suggested include dopamine blockade leading to spasm of the ischiocavernous muscles and compression of the corpora cavernosa (Pollack *et al.*, 1992). The effects of chlorpromazine on sexual function usually appear to be reversible and dose related.

Fluphenazine

Fluphenazine has been used specifically for its libido-reducing properties in sexual offenders, although paradoxically two cases of hypersexuality were reported in males treated with 12.5 mg fluphenazine decanoate every 3 weeks (Gomez, 1981).

Reduction in sexuality was found in 65 to 75% of both deviant and normal males at doses of 25 mg/day.

In a study including schizophrenic patients treated with fluphenazine, 54% of male patients reported sexual dysfunction, including erectile dysfunction and anorgasmia. Decreased quantity of ejaculate was noted in 46% (Ghadirian, Chouinard & Annable, 1982). In the same study, 30% of females reported abnormal sexual function mainly related to orgasmic difficulties.

One study looked at hormone levels in 24 male schizophrenic patients on long-term fluphenazine treatment. Two thirds had decreased libido or erectile difficulties. The prolactin levels were two to four times greater in treated patients compared with untreated healthy controls. The prolactin concentration in impotent patients tended to be higher than the non-impotent group, but the difference was not statistically significant (Arato, Erdos & Polgar, 1979).

Priapism has also been described as a complication of fluphenazine.

Perphenazine

Perphenazine caused interference with emission and ejaculation in 64% of a group of 14 patients. In some patients the effects lasted for several months after discontinuation of treatment (Buffum, 1982).

Other antipsychotics

Haloperidol. Haloperidol belongs to the butyrophenone group and as it does not produce the autonomic effects of phenothiazines it rarely produces sexual dysfunction. One case of pain on ejaculation has been reported (Berger, 1979) as has a case of impotence (Mitchell & Popkin, 1982).

Flupenthixol. A case report describes a 30-year-old schizophrenic who had experienced inability to ejaculate for several years on various neuroleptics and was latterly taking flupenthixol. This inability was reversed within a few days by the administration of cyproheptadine (see below, p. 41).

Pimozide. Pimozide is a neuroleptic belonging to the diphenyl-butylpiperidine group. It is a selective dopamine antagonist and is known to be less sedating than other compounds. A case of impotence and ejaculatory inhibition was reported at 12 to 16 mg/day (Ananth, 1982).

Trifluoperazine. Reports of interference with emission and ejaculation were shown in one early study of five patients (Blair and Simpson, 1966). Another study showed no adverse effects on ejaculation (Kotin *et al.*, 1976). Delayed female orgasm has been recorded.

Sulpiride. Sulpiride is a substituted benzamide that interacts with dopamine receptors. One study investigated prolactin levels in two groups of patients treated with sulpiride. Patients with anxiety disorders were treated with doses up to 200 mg per day and schizophrenic patients up to 600 mg per day. Patients on higher doses had higher prolactin levels. Four of the six patients taking 600 mg per day developed impotence compared with one of seven patients on the lower dose. Restoration of potency was observed after reduction or discontinuation of treatment (Weizman *et al.*, 1985). This study strongly suggests that in this group of patients the sexual side effect of the neuroleptic was related to hyperprolactinaemia.

Remoxipride. Remoxipride is a new molecule also belonging to the substituted benzamide group. It is selective for central dopaminergic receptors. No published reports of effects on sexual activity are available but the data-sheet reports menstrual disorders.

Risperidone. Risperidone is a new antipsychotic, belonging to the benzisoxazole derivatives. Erectile, ejaculatory and orgasmic dysfunction are all mentioned in the data sheet as side effects.

Clozapine. At least three recent case reports have described priapism as a complication of the new atypical antipsychotic agent clozapine.

Others. Butaperazine, chlorprothixene, mesoridazine and thiothixene have also been noted for causing sexual dysfunction. These drugs are not licensed in the UK.

Antidepressants

Sexual dysfunction is common in depression as part of the underlying disease and unfortunately most reports in the literature of sexual problems are in the form of case reports rather than controlled studies. This makes assessment of the relative contribution of the disease and the drug difficult. For example, in one study, sexual side-effects in untreated depressed patients were compared with those of a non-depressed control group (Mathew, Weinman & Claghorn, 1980). Patients were matched for age and sex. Approximately 30% of depressed patients reported one or more of the following: delayed ejaculation, premature ejaculation, impotence, loss of libido and anorgasmia. The corresponding incidence in controls was less than 10%. In addition, 20% of the depressed patients reported increased libido, which was not reported by controls.

A retrospective study (Harrison *et al.*, 1986) showed that 30% of tricyclic antidepressant-treated patients and 40% of monoamine oxidase inhibitor (MAOI)-treated patients experience some form of sexual dysfunction. The accumulated weight of evidence coupled with the mode of action of the individual drugs does lend strong support to a positive direct association between antidepressant medication and sexual dysfunction. In fact, it is believed that many antidepressants are associated with an incidence of sexual dysfunction similar to the disease itself.

Considering the number of patients on antidepressant medication, it is important to inform patients about the possibility of changes in sexual behaviour and to reassure them that these changes are reversible after cessation of treatment.

Pharmacological effects

Tricyclic antidepressants have anticholinergic properties and sympatholytic activity often responsible for causing sexual disorders. Most tricyclic antidepressants block preferentially the presynaptic reuptake of catecholamines, whereas more recent drugs such as fluoxetine or fluvoxamine are selective serotonin-reuptake inhibitors.

MAOIs increase the level of catecholamines by blocking the enzyme responsible for their degradation.

It has been suggested that brain serotonin and and catecholamine levels influence sexual activity in animals, serotonin inhibiting and catecholamines stimulating sexual behaviour.

Tricyclic antidepressants

Tricyclics antidepressants have been reported to have negative effects on several aspects of sexual function, including libido, erection, ejaculation and orgasm. Many but not all these dysfunctions can be explained by the mechanism of drug action. Erectile dysfunction may be related to increased sympathetic tone leading to constriction of the penile arteries. Ejaculatory problems could be caused by either increased noradrenaline concentrations or α-adrenoceptor blockade interfering with smooth muscle contraction in the vas and epididymis.

Imipramine

A controlled study of over 100 patients was performed by Harrison *et al.* (1986) to measure sexual dysfunction before and after treatment with imipramine or the MAOI phenelzine. Both treated males and females reported a higher incidence of sexual dysfunction than the control group. Erectile dysfunction and ejaculatory delay were reported at a daily dose of 75 mg of imipramine (Mitchell & Popkin, 1983). Decreased libido also occurred, although cases of an increase in libido have also been reported with this drug.

Clomipramine

Clomipramine is a tricyclic antidepressant that has a potent presynaptic serotonin-reuptake inhibitor activity and also inhibits noradrenaline reuptake.

One informative study exposed the weaknesses involved in the method of questioning when looking for sexual problems. Patients with an obsessive/compulsive disorder took part in a double-blind controlled study comparing clomipramine with placebo. Only a third spontaneously complained of sexual problems. The authors then performed a structured interview in all patients (7 women and 17 men) asking direct questions about sexual side effects. From this, 96% of patients who had previously been orgasmic reported anorgasmia, of which the majority had not spontaneously reported this side effect. Although a third reported decreased libido, this was felt by the patients to be secondary to anorgasmia (Monteiro *et al.*, 1987). Symptoms arose on doses as low as 25–50 mg daily.

The mechanism for anorgasmia is uncertain as it begins within days or even possibly hours of starting treatment and resolves a few days after finishing whereas the antidepressant effect takes 2 weeks to develop. Anticholinergic effects are an unlikely mechanism as high doses of anticholinergics, such as atropine, do not cause this dysfunction. Alpha-adrenergic (sympathetic) blockade is also unlikely as other α-blockers such as phenoxybenzamine cause failure of ejaculation but not anorgasmia. Another report describes reversal of clomipramine-induced anorgasmia by the administration of cyproheptadine (but not placebo) 90 minutes before anticipated sexual activity (Riley and Riley, 1986). Cyproheptadine is a serotonin (5HT) receptor antagonist, suggesting that the anorgasmia is secondary to the effect of clomipramine on serotonin activity.

A most unusual side effect of clomipramine is the occurrence of spontaneous orgasm induced by yawning. McLean and colleagues reported on a small series of patients who developed yawning on treatment. One man and one women experienced orgasm on every or most occasions when they yawned. In the male, this was associated with ejaculation. Another female patient experienced 'irresistible sexual urges' during yawning spells. There is no explanation for this phenomenon (McLean, Forsythe & Kapkin, 1983)

Other tricyclic antidepressants

Amitriptyline. Decreased libido, several cases of impotence and inhibition of ejaculation have been reported at doses of amitriptyline as low as 50 mg/day. Anorgasmia has also been reported.

Amoxapine. Decreased libido, impotence and ejaculatory inhibition have been described. One study showed that 50% of 19 males using amoxapine at doses ranging from 125 mg to 250 mg /day complained of impotence. At doses between 75 and 150 mg/day, delayed or dry ejaculation has occurred, but these effects were reversible after discontinuation of treatment.

Desipramine. There have been several cases of impotence in patients treated with desipramine. In one case report a patient developed anorgasmia on desipramine. This was successfully treated with cyproheptadine. In other cases, patients experiencing sexual dysfunction on other antidepressants benefited from switching to desipramine and found their sexual problems resolved (Buffum, 1982).

Doxepin. Decrease of libido as well as ejaculatory dysfunction were reported with doxepin (Mitchell & Popkin, 1983).

Nortriptyline. In men, case reports of impotence and ejaculatory incompetence were found at doses of nortriptyline of 75 mg/day. One case of orgasmic inhibition was also described in a woman treated with 60 mg/day (Mitchell and Popkin, 1983).

Protriptyline. Six cases of erectile dysfunction in patients taking 10 mg/day of protriptyline have been noted as well as pain on ejaculation in those taking 20 mg/day (Mitchell and Popkin, 1983).

Trimipramine. Inhibited ejaculation was described in three patients at unknown doses (Mitchell and Popkin, 1983).

Tetracyclic antidepressants

Maprotiline. Maprotiline is a tetracyclic antidepressant with similar anticholinergic effects to tricyclic compounds. Decreased libido, impotence and erectile failure were described in case reports.

Mianserin. Mianserin is a tetracyclic antidepressant with antiserotonergic properties. A double-blind study with amitriptyline and placebo showed decreased amplitude and duration of nocturnal erections in a non-psychiatric male population (Kowalski *et al.*, 1985).

Non-tricyclic antidepressants

Trazodone

This drug is a triazolopyridine antidepressant. One report describes 94 patients with abnormal erections or priapism developing as a consequence of treatment (Abber *et al.*, 1987). A few cases were irreversible and required surgery. One study showed the total duration of nocturnal erection was longer for volunteers taking trazodone compared with controls. The detumescent phase of erection was over twice as long on trazodone. Detumescence is under sympathetic control, and it is concluded that the mechanism of priapism in men is related to the α-blocking actions of trazodone interfering with sympathetic control of detumescence (Saenz de Tejada *et al.*, 1991). Male patients should, therefore, be advised to discontinue treatment should any erectile changes occur. In a few patients of both sexes, this drug has been associated with increased libido (Gartrell, 1986). The mechanism is unclear, as this effect occurs without an associated increase in mood.

Serotonin-reuptake inhibitors

Fluoxetine

Fluoxetine is a selective serotonin-reuptake inhibitor recently introduced in the USA and the UK. Since it is a relatively new compound, the sexual side-effects of the drug are mainly case reports. It has been associated with anorgasmia in both males and females. The incidence of orgasmic dysfunction described in the literature is around 8%–16% (Herman *et al.*, 1990; Musher, 1990). One patient reported ejaculatory difficulties associated with penile numbness (Neill, 1991). Jacobsen has suggested that the incidence of sexual difficulties following fluoxetine treatment is actually higher, reporting a 34% incidence of sexual dysfunction in a group of 160 treated patients (Jacobsen, 1992). These dysfunctions consisted of decreased libido and reduced sexual response and the latter category included orgasmic dysfunction and erectile disturbances. Retarded ejaculation and ejaculatory incompetence have been described in 75% of 60 patients treated in one psychiatrist's practice (Patterson, 1993). Sexual dysfunction in patients on fluoxetine was successfully treated in over 80% of patients in one study by changing to bupropion (Walker *et al.*, 1993). This drug is not available in the UK.

Intriguingly, fluoxetine has also been demonstrated to have positive effects on sexual function. In one case report, a 30-year-old woman treated with 20–60 mg/day fluoxetine experienced up to 24 spontaneous orgasms 1 hour after ingestion of fluoxetine (Modell, 1989). These episodes were preceded by sexual arousal and engorgement of the clitoris.

Also at least 30 cases of priapism have been reported to the drug manufacturer (Smith and Levitte, 1993) and geriatric patients treated with fluoxetine have developed morning erections for the first time in decades (Smith and Levitte, 1993). This has led to the suggestion that it may be used to treat erectile dysfunction, particularly in elderly patients (Power-Smith, 1994). Conversely, it has also been suggested that its effect on retarding ejaculation may be useful in the treatment of premature ejaculation (Jacobsen, 1992). Clomipramine, a tricyclic antidepressant with serotonin reuptake inhibitor properties, has also been shown in one double-blind placebo-controlled trial to be of therapeutic benefit in the treatment of premature ejaculation (Girgis, El-Haggar & El-Hermouzy, 1982).

As fluoxetine acts selectively on serotonin levels with little anticholinergic or adrenergic effect, it is tempting to speculate that the sexual effects are also mediated by serotonin. Animal data support the assumption that serotonin acting centrally is inhibitory to ejaculation. Alternatively, it may act peripherally to relax the smooth muscles of the reproductive tract involved in ejaculation and orgasm.

Fluvoxamine

Fluvoxamine was the first serotonin-reuptake inhibitor introduced in the antidepressant spectrum. Two recent case reports have described anorgasmia and erectile and ejaculatory failure occurring in three patients following initiation of fluvoxamine therapy (Dorevitch and Davis, 1994).

Sertraline and paroxetine

These two drugs are new serotonin-reuptake inhibitors recently introduced in the UK. In a placebo-and amitriptyline-controlled study assessing sertraline, there was a higher incidence of male sexual dysfunction in sertraline-treated patients than in the two control groups (Reimherr *et al.*, 1990). One report quoting drug company placebo-controlled studies gave an incidence of sexual dysfunction of 17% for patients on sertraline and 3% on paroxetine (Grimsley & Jann, 1992).

Monoamine oxidase inhibitors

Drugs with MAOI activity are often used when other antidepressants have failed. Older literature suggests that they produce sexual dysfunction in 10–30%. In a placebo-controlled trial, Harrison found that 40% of 35 patients taking phenelzine had decreased sexual function including reduced libido and anorgasmia (Harrison *et al.*, 1986). In this study, the sexual effects of *phenelzine* were more pronounced than those of the tricyclic antidepressant imipramine. Several case reports have described anorgasmia as a complication of treatment with phenelzine (Lesko, Stotland & Segraves, 1982). In a large study of 198 patients on antidepressants,

Rabkin *et al.* (1985) found that 22% of 141 patients on phenelzine experienced complete anorgasmia or impotence. Others with less marked degrees of sexual dysfunction, such as reduced libido or delayed sexual response, were excluded, so the total percentage with sexual side effects was higher. In this same study, only 2% of 41 patients taking *tranylcypromine* had anorgasmia or impotence.

One report has described spontaneous improvement of phenelzine-induced anorgasmia despite continuation of treatment in three patients (Nurnberg & Levine, 1987).

Lithium

Lithium is used in a large number of manic-depressive patients, but the incidence of quoted sexual side effects is difficult to establish. The incidence is probably low (approximately 5 to 10%), but some older studies did report sexual dysfunction in up to 50% of patients. The main sexual disturbances described are reduced libido and erectile dysfunction. Difficulties in evaluating manic-depressive patients arise because there is a tendency to hypersexuality during manic episodes. In contrast to this, the reduced sexual desires experienced during treatment may be considered by the patient to be abnormally low libido whereas it may just be an expression of the therapeutic effect of the drug. Also lithium can provoke hypothyroidism, which in itself can be a cause of sexual dysfunction.

In a Canadian study, 14% of patients receiving lithium alone experienced sexual difficulties (Gharidian *et al.* 1992). The percentage increases to nearly 50% when lithium is combined with benzodiazepines. There is a possibility that lithium potentiates the sexual side effects of these compounds. The effects reported are mainly decreased libido, erectile dysfunction and delayed ejaculation in men.

A retrospective Danish study (Kristensen & Jørgensen, 1987) showed no difference in any aspect of sexual function between treated patients and untreated controls but the potentiation of sexual effects caused by combination therapy is also mentioned.

Treatment of antidepressant-induced sexual dysfunction

Sexual dysfunction appears to be a frequent problem for patients on antidepressants. The easiest management of sexual problems caused by antidepressant treatment is to substitute the medication for another drug less likely to provoke these effects. For example, switching from imipramine to desipramine relieved sexual disturbances in one report (Sovner, 1983). However, if the drug is of therapeutic benefit, the patient may not wish to change to another drug but would nevertheless appreciate treatment of any sexual dysfunction. As the patient's mood improves, this may be associated with an increase in sexual desire. If this is accompanied by sexual dysfunction, it can become a source of frustration.

Several drugs have been used to treat antidepressant-induced sexual dysfunction.

Cyproheptadine

As discussed earlier, the serotonin receptor antagonist cyproheptadine reverses clomipramine-induced anorgasmia (Riley and Riley, 1986). Another report showed that it also improved anorgasmia provoked by fluoxetine (McCormick, Olin & Brotman, 1990). Recently, cyproheptadine has been used to reverse anorgasmia provoked by fluvoxamine (Arnott & Nutt, 1994). Cyproheptadine also successfully reversed inability to ejaculate in one schizophrenic man on flupenthixol. The report did not mention whether he experienced orgasm on flupenthixol. However, after treatment he was able to resume 'pleasurable ejaculation' (Jeffries & Walker, 1987).

In one case report, anorgasmia developed from desipramine therapy. This was successfully treated with cyproheptadine. This patient developed an anticholinergic crisis on cyproheptadine, associated with tachycardia, hypertension and a fever. Although a serotonin blocker, cyproheptadine also has weak anticholinergic activity, which was thought to act synergistically with desipramine to induce the crisis (Pontius, 1988). Another potential danger is that the addition of cyproheptadine reverses not only the sexual dysfunction but also the therapeutic benefit, causing a relapse of depressive symptoms. This is particularly true for antidepressants that act as serotonin-reuptake inhibitors. (Goldbloom & Kennedy, 1991).

Bethanecol

Bethanecol is a peripheral cholinergic drug that has been successfully used to reverse impotence in men and anorgasmia in women taking tranylcypromine, isocarboxazid and amoxapine (Gross, 1982) as well as some tricyclic antidepressants (Yager, 1986). It is presumed to act by opposing the anticholinergic effects of antidepressants although, as there is evidence that it also reverses ejaculatory problems, the action may be more complex than this (Sorscher & Dilsaver, 1986).

Yohimbine

The sexual side effects of clomipramine have successfully been treated with yohimbine in five patients (Hollander & McCarley, 1992). This is predominantly an α_2-adrenergic antagonist and possibly acts centrally as the penis has predominantly α_1-adrenoceptors (Price and Grunhaus, 1990). Jacobsen (1992) reported that eight of nine patients with fluoxetine-induced sexual dysfunction responded to yohimbine.

Amantadine

One study showed that fluoxetine-induced anorgasmia was reversed in two of four patients treated with amantadine, a dopamine agonist (Balogh, Hendricks & Kang, 1992). This supports animal studies, which have suggested that serotonin inhibits while dopamine facilitates ejaculation.

Anxiolytics

Benzodiazepines

Benzodiazepines have been associated with decreased libido, anorgasmia, erectile dysfunction and inability to achieve ejaculation. Most published reports concern alprazolam.

Alprazolam

A series of case reports have described decreased libido in both men and women, anorgasmia in women and inhibition of ejaculation in men following short-term treatment with alprazolam. These side effects were reversed shortly after discontinuing treatment. In one study, 32 patients on alprazolam for anxiety disorders completed a questionnaire comparing their sexual function after several weeks of treatment with their pre-drug function. Fifty per cent reported decreased libido and a similar percentage described their ability to achieve orgasm as much worse than before starting the drug. Four of nine men recorded erectile difficulties, including one man who was unable to achieve erection. A small percentage of patients noted an improvement in sexual function on therapy. The authors found that reducing the drug dose or changing medication reduced or reversed unwanted sexual side effects (Lydiard *et al.*, 1987).

Chlordiazepoxide

Ejaculatory incompetence was reported in one man taking 20 mg/day.

Clonazepam

Occasional cases of anorgasmia in females and impaired erectile function in males have been described following the use of clonazepam in the treatment of panic disorders. In the cases cited, normal sexual function was regained when the dose of clonazepam was reduced (Cohen and Rosenbaum, 1987).

Diazepam

Decreased libido and problems with erection have been reported in two men taking diazepam at doses of 25 and 40 mg/day, respectively. Neither was sedated and normal sexual function returned following a change to another benzodiazepine, clonazepam. (Balon, Ramesh & Pohl, 1989).

Lorazepam

In two case reports, lorazepam has been implicated in causing delayed ejaculation and complete loss of libido with short-term use at doses of 1–3 mg/day. Normal sexual function returned within 1 week of cessation of treatment (Khandelwal, 1988). Lorazepam has also been used in the treatment of premature ejaculation.

Antiepileptics

Sexual dysfunction in epilepsy

Lack of interest in sex is a very common finding in epileptic patients, it is reported in 33 to 66% of men and 14 to 50% of women. Most of these figures are based on retrospective data, which depend on the patient's long-term memory. This may be a problem for some epileptic patients. Two studies have quantitatively assessed sexual function in epileptics. One showed decreased nocturnal penile tumescence in men. The other looked at penile and vaginal blood flow in response to erotic visual stimulation. Both epileptic patients and healthy controls reported the same degree of subjective sexual arousal, indicating similar libido, but blood flow to the genital areas was significantly reduced in the epileptic group, illustrating a dissociation between libido and potency.

Several factors have been proposed to explain hyposexuality in epilepsy. It may be a consequence of an altered social or emotional development, particularly relating to poor self esteem or an association between sexual arousal and seizure activity. Alternatively, as sexual dysfunction usually only arises after the onset of seizure activity, a direct effect of the epileptic discharges on the limbic system in the hypothalamus has been suggested. Furthermore, there is clear evidence that epilepsy is associated with disturbances of the hypothalamic-pituitary axis, affecting both gonadotrophin and prolactin secretion. For example, prolactin levels rise markedly shortly after a seizure. Finally, the role of antiepileptic drugs themselves in producing sexual disturbances needs to be considered (Mattson & Cramer, 1985; Morrell, 1991).

Reproductive effects of antiepileptic drugs

Effect on hormones

A large number of epileptic patients are treated with more than one antiepileptic drug at a time. Many of the studies assessing the influence of medication have not been able to correlate effects with specific drugs or, if they have, only a few patients have been available for investigation. Results are sometimes variable between different studies but the following changes appear to be the most consistent.

Sex hormone-binding globulin (SHBG) levels are increased, which leads to a reduction in the level of free testosterone (Victor, Lundberg & Johansson, 1977; Toone, Wheeler & Fenwick, 1980). Total testosterone levels (which includes both free hormone and that bound to proteins such as SHBG) are either normal or elevated. LH levels are usually significantly increased (Toone *et al.,* 1983; Macphee *et al.,* 1988). Toone and co-workers (1983) were able to correlate the reduction in free testosterone level to two aspects of sexual drive, namely the frequency of early morning erections and sexual activity leading to orgasm.

There are two explanations for the hormone abnormalities seen. One possibility is that antiepileptic drugs induce liver enzymes thereby increasing the production of SHBG. This binds more testosterone, reducing the amount of biologically active free testosterone. Pituitary LH is secreted in greater amounts to try to increase testicular testosterone production. Alternatively, it is possible that the primary abnormality is a reduction in free testosterone as a consequence of increased metabolism. This leads to a rise in LH to increase testosterone synthesis, accompanied by a secondary rise in SHBG (Toone *et al.* 1983).

Macphee *et al.* (1988) noted that untreated epileptics had hormone levels similar to healthy controls. They investigated hormone concentrations in epileptics taking *carbamazepine, phenytoin* and *sodium valproate* as well as patients taking multiple drug combinations. Patients on multiple drugs had abnormalities of all hormones measured, including raised

SHBG, reduced free testosterone and high LH levels. In contrast, drugs used individually only appeared to have isolated actions. For example, carbamazepine was associated with reduced free testosterone levels and high LH but normal SHBG. Phenytoin, however, caused a significant increase in SHBG levels without a significant effect on free testosterone. It should be noted that in three of the thirteen patients on phenytoin, free testosterone levels were below the lowest of the 40 control patients. Sodium valproate had no effect on any of the hormones measured. It follows that different antiepileptic drugs exert their effects via different mechanisms. Carbamazepine had no effect on SHBG levels; therefore, it probably reduces testosterone by increased hepatic clearance of testosterone. For phenytoin, increased SHBG synthesis may be the more important mechanism. This study did demonstrate that sodium valproate may be a good alternative treatment for male epileptic patients with sexual dysfunction.

Whether these hormone changes are sufficient to explain the reduced sexual function in epileptic patients is uncertain. For example, in one study in men, decreased libido and potency were more often reported with use of *phenobarbitone* or *primidone* than with phenytoin or carbamazepine, despite the fact that all four drugs are potent inducers of liver enzymes (Mattson *et al.*, 1985).

Less information is available on the effect of epilepsy on female reproductive function. It is recognised that in some women the frequency of epileptic seizures is higher in the late follicular phase when oestrogen levels are high and reduced in the mid-luteal phase when progesterone levels are maximal. There have been some studies which suggest that women with epilepsy are more likely to have irregular menstrual cycles linked to anovulation, but gonadotrophin levels were not measured to assess if this was an ovarian or hypothalamic-pituitary effect. The fertility of epileptic women has not been directly studied.

Effect on sperm

Epileptic patients often receive long-term medication and combined antiepileptics. Toone and co-workers (1983) suggested that long-term treatment may lead to testicular failure and impaired spermatogenesis. Alterations to sperm parameters, including motility, were first described in 1975, but only a few studies have tried to investigate this in more detail. It has been suggested that as antiepileptic drugs suppress neuronal irritability by stabilising cell membranes they may also have an adverse effect on sperm membranes. One study assessed sperm parameters in a group of 10 epileptics receiving long-term medication. Five were taking phenytoin alone and the others were receiving multiple therapy. Sperm motility was quantified by assessing the ability of the sperm to migrate across a micropore membrane. Motility measured in this way was significantly reduced in the treated epileptic patients compared with healthy donors. The authors also performed an *in vitro* study in which the motility of donor sperm was assessed after addition of high concentrations of antiepileptic drugs to the sperm preparation. The drugs did adversely affect sperm motility *in vitro* but only at concentrations much higher than those found in the clinical context. The authors noted that they were only looking at acute exposure, whereas treated epileptics are chronically exposed to these drugs (Chen *et al.*, 1992).

A recent study has looked at conventional sperm parameters in untreated epileptics, epileptics treated with long-term phenytoin and healthy controls (Taneja *et al.*, 1994). Interestingly, semen volume was reduced in both treated and untreated epileptic patients. Both these groups also showed significant reductions in sperm concentration compared with controls. There was no difference between treated and untreated epileptic patients. These results raise the possibility that fertility may be reduced in epileptic patients irrespective of treatment, although there is no direct evidence for this in the literature. It has been suggested that the apparent reduction of fertility in epileptic men may be related to hyposexuality and the absence of a sexual partner.

New anticonvulsants

No information is available concerning potential reproductive effects of the newer anticonvulsants, i.e. the gamma-aminobutyric acid (GABA) analogues such as *vigabatrin*, which inhibits GABA transaminase, and *gabapentin*. These drugs are not hepatic enzyme inducers. *Lamotrigine* inhibits the release of glutamate.

It is probably still too early to know if these drugs have adverse effects on sexual function.

Antiparkinsonians

Levodopa

Levodopa is usually used in the treatment of Parkinson's disease, which occurs more frequently in elderly patients and, therefore, sexual side effects are less likely to come to light. One early report did describe the use of levodopa to treat three middle-aged psychiatric patients (diagnosis not specified). Two of them complained that, following treatment, they experienced lack of ejaculation during intercourse despite normal erection and orgasm (Hällström & Persson, 1970).

In Parkinson's disease, the influence of levodopa on sexual function is variable. In general, approximately 50% of men being treated with levodopa for parkinsonism report improved sexual interest or activity. In one study, the increased sexual interest was associated in some patients with raised baseline LH levels, which presumably would increase testosterone production, although this was not measured (Brown *et al.*, 1978).

Bromocriptine

The sexual side effects of bromocriptine are discussed in Chapter 5.

Other central nervous system drugs

Cinnarizine

Cinnarizine is a calcium-channel blocker used for migraine prophylaxis, dizziness, vertigo and motion sickness. It has a prominent dopamine antagonist effect. A recent case report has described erectile impotence occurring 3 months after initiation of cinnarizine treatment, which resolved within 3 days of stopping the drug. The effect was believed to be caused by the antidopaminergic activity (Sempere *et al.*, 1993).

References

Abber, J. C., Lue, T. F., Luo, J. A., Juenemann, K. P. & Tanagho, E. A. (1987) Priapism induced by chlorpromazine and trazodone: mechanism of action. *Journal of Urology*, 137, 1039–42.

Ananth, J. (1982). Impotence associated with pimozide. *American Journal of Psychiatry*, 139, 1374.

Arato, M., Erdos, A. & Polgar, M. (1979). Endocrinological changes in patients with sexual dysfunction under long-term neuroleptic treatment. *Pharmakopsychiatrie Neuro-psychopharmakologie*, 12, 426–31.

Arnott, S. & Nutt, D. (1994). Successful treatment of fluvoxamine-induced anorgasmia by cyproheptadine. *British Journal of Psychiatry*, 164, 838–9.

Balogh, S., Hendricks, S. E. & Kang, J. (1992). Treatment of fluoxetine-induced anorgasmia with amantadine. *Journal of Clinical Psychiatry*, 53, 212–13.

Balon, R., Ramesh, C. & Pohl, R. (1989). Sexual dysfunction associated with diazepam but not clonazepam. *Canadian Journal of Psychiatry*, 9, 947–8.

Berger, S. M. (1979). Trifluoroperazine and haloperidol: sources of ejaculatory pain. *American Journal of Psychiatry*, 136, 350.

Blair, J. & Simpson, G. (1966). Effects of antipsychotic drugs on reproductive functions. *Diseases of the Nervous System*, 27, 645–7.

Brown, E., Brown, G. M., Kofman, O. & Quarrington, B. (1978). Sexual function and affect in Parkinsonian men treated with L-dopa. *American Journal of Psychiatry*, 135, 1552–5.

Brown, W. A., Laughren, T. & Williams, B. (1981). Differential effects of neuroleptic agents on the pituitary-gonadal axis in men. *Archives of general Psychiatry*, 38, 1270–2

Buffum, J. (1982). Pharmacosexology:the effects of drugs on sexual function – a review. *Journal of Psychoactive Drugs*, 14, 5–44.

Buffum, J. (1986). Pharmacosexology update: prescription drugs and sexual function. *Journal of Psychoactive Drugs*, 18, 97–106.

Chen, S.-S., Shen, M.-R., Chen, T.-J. & Lai, S.-L. (1992). Effects of antiepileptic drugs on sperm motility of normal controls and epileptic patients with long-term therapy. *Epilepsia*, 33, 149–53.

Chen, Y. H. & Lee, A. S. (1990). Neuroleptic-induced priapism, hepatotoxicity and subsequent impotence in a patient with depressive psychosis. *British Journal of Psychiatry*, 157, 759–62.

Cohen, L. S. & Rosenbaum, J. F. (1987). Clonazepam: new uses and potential problems. *Journal of Clinical Psychiatry*, 48 (suppl.), 50–6.

Dorevitch, A. & Davis, H. (1994). Fluvoxamine-associated sexual dysfunction. *Annals of Pharmacotherapy*, 28, 872–4.

Gartrell, N. (1986). Increased libido in women receiving trazodone. *American Journal of Psychiatry*, 143, 781–2.

Ghadirian, A.-M., Chouinard, G. & Annable, L. (1982). Sexual dysfunction and plasma prolactin levels in neuroleptic-treated schizophrenic outpatients. *Journal of Nervous and Mental Disease*, 170, 463–7.

Ghadirian, A.-M., Annable, L. & Bélanger, M.-C. (1992). Lithium, benzodiazepines and sexual function in bipolar patients. *American Journal of Psychiatry*, 149, 801–5.

Girgis, S. M., El-Haggar, S. & El-Hermouzy, S. (1982). A double-blind trial of clomipramine in premature ejaculation. *Andrologia*, 14, 364–8.

Goldbloom, D. S. & Kennedy, S. H. (1991). Adverse interaction of fluoxetine and cyproheptadine in two patients with bulimia nervosa. *Journal of Clinical Psychiatry*, 52, 261–2.

Gomez, E. A. (1981). Hypersexuality in men receiving fluphenazine decanoate. *American Journal of Psychiatry*, 138, 1263.

Grimsley, S. R. & Jann, M. W. (1992). Paroxetine, sertraline, and fluvoxamine: new selective serotonin reuptake inhibitors. *Clinical Pharmacy*, 11, 930–57.

Gross, M. D. (1982). Reversal by bethanecol of sexual dysfunction caused by anticholinergic antidepressants. *American Journal of Psychiatry*, 139, 1193–4.

Hällström, T. & Persson, T. (1970). L-dopa and non-emission of semen. *Lancet*, 1231–2.

Harrison, W. M., Rabkin, J. G., Ehrhardt, A. A., Stewart, J. W., McGrath, P. J., Ross, D. & Quitkin, F. M. (1986). Effects of antidepressant medication on sexual function: a controlled study. *Journal of Clinical Psychopharmacology*, 6, 144–9.

Herman, J. B., Brotman, A. W., Pollack, M. H., Falk, W. E., Biederman, J. & Rosenbaum, J. F. (1990). Fluoxetine-induced sexual dysfunction. *Journal of Clinical Psychiatry*, 51, 25–7.

Hollander, E. & McCarley, A. (1992). Yohimbine treatment of sexual side effects induced by serotonin reuptake inhibitors. *Journal of Clinical Psychiatry*, 53, 207–9.

Jackson, S. C. & Walker, J. S. (1991). Self administered intraurethral chlorpromazine: an unusual cause of priapism. *American Journal of Emergency Medicine*, 9, 171–5.

Jacobsen, F. M. (1992). Fluoxetine-induced sexual dysfunction and an open trial of yohimbine. *Journal of Clinical Psychiatry*, 53, 119–22.

Jeffries, J. J. & Walker, C. (1987). Cyproheptadine and drug-induced anorgasmia. *Canadian Journal of Psychiatry*, 32, 79.

Khandelwal, S. K. (1988). Complete loss of libido with short-term use of lorazepam. *American Journal of Psychiatry*, 145, 1313–14.

Kotin, J., Wilbert, D. E., Verburg, D. & Soldinger, S. M. (1976). Thioridazine and sexual function. *American Journal of Psychiatry*, 133, 82–5.

Kowalski, A., Stanley, R. O., Dennerstein, L, Burrows, G. & Maguire, K. P. (1985). The sexual side effects of antidepressant medication: a double-blind comparison of two antidepressants in a non-psychiatric population. *British Journal of Psychiatry*, 147, 413–18.

Kristensen, E. & Jørgensen, P. (1987). Sexual function in lithium-treated manic-depressive patients. *Pharmacopsychiatry*, 20, 165–7.

Lesko, L. M., Stotland, N. L. & Segraves, R. T. (1982). Three cases of anorgasmia associated with MAOIs. *American Journal of Psychiatry*, 139, 1353–4.

Lydiard, R. B., Howell, E. F., Laraia, M. T. & Ballenger, J. C. (1987). Sexual side effects of alprazolam. *American Journal of Psychiatry*, 144, 254–5.

Macphee, G. J. A., Larkin, J. G., Butler, E., Beastall, G. H. & Brodie, M. J. (1988). Circulating hormones and pituitary responsiveness in young epileptic men receiving long-term antiepileptic medication. *Epilepsia*, 29, 468–75.

Mathew, R. J., Weinman, M. & Claghorn, J. L. (1980). Tricyclic side effects without tricyclics in depression. *Psychopharmamacology Bulletin*, 16, 58–60.

Mattson, R. H. & Cramer, J. A. (1985). Epilepsy, sex hormones, and antiepileptic drugs. *Epilepsia*, 26 (suppl) S40–S51.

Mattson, R. H., Cramer, J. A., Collins, J. F., Smith, D. B., Delgado-Escueta, A. V., Browne, T. R., Williamson, P. D., Treiman, D. M., McNamara, J. O., McCutchen, C. B., Homa, R. W., Crill, W. E., Lubozynski, M. F., Rosenthal, N. P. & Mayersdorf, A. (1985). Comparison of carbamazepine, phenobarbital, phenytoin, and primidone in partial and secondarily generalised tonic–clonic seizures. *New England Journal of Medicine*, 313, 145–51.

McCormick, S., Olin, J. & Brotman, A. W. (1990). Reversal of fluoxetine-induced anorgasmia by cyproheptadine in two patients. *Journal of Clinical Psychiatry*, 51, 383–4.

McLean, J. D., Forsythe, R. G. & Kapkin, I. A. (1983). Unusual side effects of clomipramine associated with yawning. *Canadian Journal of Psychiatry*, 28, 569–70.

Mitchell, J. E. & Popkin, M. K. (1982). Antipsychotic drug therapy and sexual dysfunction in men. *American Journal of Psychiatry*, 139, 633–7.

Mitchell, J. E. & Popkin, M. K. (1983). Antidepressant drug therapy and sexual dysfunction in men: a review. *Journal of Clinical Psychopharmacology*, 3, 76–9.

Modell, J. G. (1989). Repeated observations of yawning, clitoral engorgement and orgasm associated with fluoxetine administration. *Journal of Clinical Psychopharmacology*, 9, 63–5.

Monteiro, W. O., Noshirvani, H. F., Marks, I. M. & Lelliott, P. T. (1987). Anorgasmia from clomipramine in obsessive-compulsive disorder: a controlled trial. *British Journal of Psychiatry*, 151, 107–12.

Morrell, M. J. (1991). Sexual dysfunction in epilepsy. *Epilepsia*, 32 (suppl.), S38–S45.

Musher, J. S. (1990). Anorgasmia with the use of fluoxetine. *American Journal of Psychiatry*, 147, 948.

Neill, J. R. (1991). Penile anesthesia associated with fluoxetine use. *American Journal of Psychiatry*, 148, 1603.

Nestoros, J. N., Lehmann, H. E. & Ban, T. A. (1981). Sexual behaviour of the male schizophrenic: the impact of illness and medications. *Archives of Sexual Behaviour*, 10, 421–42.

Nurnberg, H. G. & Levine, P. E. (1987). Spontaneous remission of MAOI-induced anorgasmia. *American Journal of Psychiatry*, 144, 805–7.

Patterson, W. M. (1993). Fluoxetine-induced sexual dysfunction. *Journal of Clinical Psychiatry*, 54, 71.

Pollack, M. H., Reiter, S. & Hammerness, P. (1992). Genitourinary and sexual adverse effects of psychotropic medication. *International Journal of Psychiatry in Medicine*, 22, 305–27.

Pontius, E. B. (1988). Case report of an anticholinergic crisis associated with cyproheptadine treatment of desipramine-induced inorgasmia. *Journal of Clinical Psychopharmacology*, 8, 230–1.

Power-Smith, P. (1994). Beneficial sexual side-effects from fluoxetine. *British Journal of Psychiatry*. 164, 249–50.

Price, J. & Grunhaus, L. J. (1990). Treatment of clomipramine-induced anorgasmia with yohimbine: a case report. *Journal of Clinical Psychiatry*, 51, 32–3.

Rabkin, J. G., Quitkin, F. M., McGrath, P., Harrison, W. & Tricamo, E. (1985). Adverse reactions to monoamine oxidase inhibitors. Part II. Treatment correlates and clinical management. *Journal of Clinical Psychopharmacology*, 5, 2–9.

Reimherr, F. W., Chouinard, G., Cohn, C. K., Cole, J. O., Itil, T. M., LaPierre, Y. D., Masco, H. L. & Mendels, J. (1990). Antidepressant efficacy of sertraline: a double-blind, placebo- and amitriptyline-controlled, multicentre comparison study in outpatients with major depression. *Journal of Clinical Psychiatry*, 51 (suppl. B), 18–27.

Riley, A. J. & Riley, E. J. (1986). Cyproheptadine and antidepressant-induced anorgasmia. *British Journal of Psychiatry*, 148, 217–18.

Saenz de Tejada, I., Ware, J. C., Blanco, R., Pittard, J. T., Nadig, P. W., Azadzoi, K. M., Krane, R. J. & Goldstein, I. (1991). Pathology of prolonged penile erection associated with trazodone use. *Journal of Urology*, 145, 60–4.

Sandison, R. A., Whitelaw, E. & Currie, J. D. (1960). Clinical trials with Melleril (TP21). *Journal of Mental Science*, 106, 732–41.

Sempere, A. P., Garcia, F. M., Duarte, J., Mataix, A. L., Coria, F. & Claverai, L. E. (1993). Impotence associated with cinnarizine. *Annals of Pharmacotherapy*, 27, 370–1.

Shader, R. (1964). Sexual dysfunction associated with thioridazine hydrochloride. *Journal of the American Medical Association*, 188, 1007–9.

Shen, W. W. & Park, S. (1982). Thioridazine-induced inhibition of female orgasm. *Psychiatric Journal of the University of Ottawa*, 7, 249–51.

Smith, D. M. & Levitte, S. S. (1993). Association of fluoxetine and return of sexual potency in three elderly men. *Journal of Clinical Psychiatry*, 54, 317–19.

Sorscher, S. M. & Dilsaver, S. C. (1986). Antidepressant-induced sexual dysfunction in men: due to cholinergic blockade? *Journal of Clinical Psychopharmacology*, 6, 53–5.

Sovner, R. (1983). Anorgasmia associated with imipramine but not desipramine: case report. *Journal of Clinical Psychiatry*, 44, 345–6.

Taneja, N., Kucheria, K., Jain, S. & Maheshwari, M. C. (1994). Effect of phenytoin on sperm. *Epilepsia*, 35, 136–40.

Toone, B. K., Wheeler, M. & Fenwick, P. B. C. (1980). Sex hormone changes in male epileptics. *Clinical Endocrinology*, 12, 391–5.

Toone, B. K., Wheeler, M. Nanjee, M., Fenwick, P. & Grant, R. (1983). Sex hormones, sexual activity and plasma anticonvulsant levels in male epileptics. *Journal of Neurology, Neurosurgery, and Psychiatry*, 46, 824–6.

Victor, A., Lundberg, P. O. & Johansson, E. D. (1977). Induction of sex hormone binding globulin by phenytoin. *British Medical Journal*, 2, 934–5.

Walker. P. W., Cole, J. O., Gardner, E. A., Hughes, A. R., Johnston, J. A., Batey, S. R. & Lineberry, C. G. (1993). Improvement in fluoxetine-associated sexual function in patients switched to bupropion. *Journal of Clinical Psychiatry*, 54, 459–69.

Weizman, A., Maoz, B., Treves, I., Asher, I. & Ben-David, M. (1985). Sulpiride-induced hyperprolactinaemia and impotence in male psychiatric outpatients. *Progress in Neuro-Psychopharmacology and Biological Psychiatry*, 9, 193–8.

Yager, J. (1986). Bethanecol chloride can reverse erectile and ejaculatory dysfunction induced by tricyclic antidepressants and mazindol: case report. *Journal of Clinical Psychiatry*, 47, 210–11.

4

Cancer chemotherapy

Factors influencing reproductive toxicity

Chemotherapeutic agents can have significant toxic effects on the gonads and these cause major degrees of reproductive dysfunction. In the early days of cancer chemotherapy, reproductive toxicity was a secondary consideration to attempting to cure the disease. Fertility only became a concern when cancer treatment was associated with disease remission and patient survival. Now that some cancers are 100% curable, future reproductive capacity is of major importance to patients, particularly young men and women. Patients may only agree to chemotherapy that does not harm their ability to become parents.

Early cancer chemotherapy usually consisted of the administration of a single drug, and identification of the agent responsible for reproductive toxicity was obvious. Significant information is available from early studies and follow-up data are now available to assess the possibility of long-term recovery of reproductive function following treatment. More recent trends in cancer chemotherapy are towards combinations of several cytotoxic drugs with different mechanisms of action. The aim is to maximise cytotoxic activity while reducing toxicity to healthy tissues. Consequently, it is often less apparent which of the drugs used is responsible for the toxic effect.

In general, cytotoxic drugs exert the most marked effect on rapidly dividing tissue, and germ cells are particularly sensitive. The reproductive consequence of the treatment depends not only on the dose administered but also the sex of the patient and the stage in reproductive life. The neoplastic process itself may also adversely affect sexual function.

This chapter will review the mechanisms of action of cytotoxic therapy and describe known associated reproductive toxicity. There are separate sections for drug effects in adult men, adult women, prepubertal

Table 4.1. *Drugs classified as alkylating agents*

Cyclophosphamide
Ifosfamide
Mustine (nitrogen mustard, mechlorethamine)
Busulphan
Chlorambucil
Melphelan
Carmustine

and pubertal children, where the data are available. The effect of cytotoxics on gametes differs in the two sexes, reflecting the time course necessary for the development of mature gametes from the primitive germ cells. In adult men, the formation of mature spermatozoa from primitive germ cells occurs over a 60 to 90 day cycle. In women, mitotic proliferation of the primitive germ cells to ova occurs in fetal life. The first meiotic division also begins at this time and then oocyte development is arrested until 24 to 48 hours before ovulation. Some ova are held in this arrested state for more than 40 years. Chemotherapeutic agents that damage rapidly dividing cells are, therefore, more likely to influence men than women.

Alkylating agents

Alkylating agents inhibit DNA synthesis by binding to specific DNA bases and inactivating the DNA template. This effect occurs in resting cells, but abnormal reading of the DNA code by RNA leads to disordered protein synthesis, resulting in damage to rapidly dividing cells as well (Damewood and Grochow 1986).

A list of alkylating agents is shown in Table 4.1. In the following sections, those alkylating agents that have been most extensively investigated will be discussed, although it is probable that all alkylating agents will have similar reproductive toxicity.

Effects in adult men

Cyclophosphamide

Nitrogen mustard, the earliest alkylating agent, was recorded as being toxic to the testis in 1948 when autopsy studies showed absent spermatogenesis in 90% of a group of 30 men being treated for lymphoma (Spitz 1948). The toxic effects of cyclophosphamide on testicular and reproductive function were not fully recognised until 1972 (Fairley, Barrie & Johnson, 1972). This has since been confirmed in many studies for both cyclophosphamide and chlorambucil. A progressive decline in sperm numbers resulting in azoospermia is seen within 3 to 4 months of commencing daily cyclophosphamide. At light microscopy, the damage is seen to be confined to the germinal epithelium with sparing of Leydig cells. Raised plasma FSH and LH occur, although testosterone concentrations remain normal.

Age at the time of treatment is a significant factor in determining toxicity. The testicular effect, both short and long term, is dose dependent. Men treated with a total dose of cyclophosphamide in excess of 18 g develop azoospermia (Chapman, 1983). Conversely at daily doses of 2 to 4.6 mg/kg for less than 2 months, normal testicular function was retained (Etteldorf *et al.*, 1976).

There is often partial recovery of spermatogenesis following cyclophosphamide therapy. A recent study in men treated with cyclophosphamide as part of a combination regimen for sarcomas found recovery from azoospermia to normal levels occurred in 70% of patients receiving doses less than 7.5 g/m^2 but only in 10% of those receiving doses exceeded 7.5 g/m^2. Few patients showed recovery after 5 years of azoospermia (Meistrich *et al.*, 1992).

Chlorambucil

Azoospermia developed in men treated for lymphoma following a total dose of 400 mg of chlorambucil. Typically there is a progressive decline to azoospermia within 2 to 3 months of therapy. Testicular biopsies in these patients showed germinal aplasia with normal appearances of Sertoli and Leydig cells (Schilsky *et al.*, 1980). Plasma FSH may be normal or increased. Spermatogenesis may return a long time after discontinuation of chlorambucil. A recent French report describes two men treated with chlorambucil. One received a total dose of between 5400 and 6500 mg. Six years later he was azoospermic with high plasma FSH levels. Fifteen years later spermatogenesis returned and 19 years after treatment the sperm count was normal. Another man received a dose of between 3000 and 4400 mg of chlorambucil. Fourteen years later he was also azoospermic with raised FSH. Nineteen years after treatment a normal sperm count was recorded (Marmor *et al.*, 1992).

Estramustine

This drug, a combination of an oestrogen and the alkylating agent mustine, is used for prostatic cancer. In one study, all patients treated developed loss of libido (Johansson *et al.*, 1987).

Effects in adult women

Monitoring the effects of chemotherapeutic drugs in women is more diffi-cult than in men as there is no direct way of measuring the toxic effect on the gametes (oocytes). Only indirect information is available from changes in the menstrual cycle or assessment of serum hormone levels (in earlier studies urinary hormone levels were used to gauge drug-induced damage to the ovary).

Typically gonadal damage is manifest in women by amenorrhoea accompanied by low oestrogen levels and raised concentrations of the gonadotrophins FSH and LH. This is the classical hormonal picture nor-mally seen at the menopause. Several investigators have biopsied the ovaries of affected women and confirmed the depletion of oocytes. Warne examined ovarian biopsies from cyclophosphamide-treated patients and noted the absence of oocytes and their surrounding cells. There was no evidence of any degree of maturation of the ovarian follicles (Warne *et al.*, 1973).

Busulphan

In 1960, busulphan was the first cytotoxic to be reported to affect ovarian function, producing amenorrhoea in women being treated for chronic myelogenous leukaemia. Early studies showed the amenorrhoea to be irre-versible in patients receiving doses of 0.5 to 14 mg/day busulphan for 3 months. This was followed by other reports describing amenorrhoea and menopausal symptoms in women treated with chlorambucil and cyclophosphamide (see Chapman, 1984 for review).

Cyclophosphamide and chlorambucil

Amenorrhoea induced by cyclophosphamide is irreversible in over 90% of patients, although younger women treated for short periods have the best hope for resumption of ovarian activity. There appears to be both age and sex differences in the gonadal effect of alkylating agents. Females receiving high doses of cyclophosphamide, sufficient to cause irreversible azoo-spermia in men, report a lesser influence on ovarian function with the possibility of a resumption of fertility. The age factor presumably relates to the size of the residual pool of oocytes, as the dose of cyclophosphamide necessary to induce amenorrhoea is 5.2 g in those over 40 years, 9.3 g in patients in their thirties and 20.4 g for those in their twenties (Shalet, 1980).

Damage to the ovaries may be progressive. Pregnancies have been recorded in women with ovarian dysfunction secondary to chemotherapy. Some of these women have subsequently gone on to develop premature ovarian failure. At birth, there are approximately 2 million ovarian primordial follicles. This number is progressively depleted throughout reproductive life so that ovarian failure occurs physiologically at the natural menopause when the pool of ovarian follicles has reduced to approximately 400. Cytotoxic-induced ovarian damage, insufficient to provoke immediate ovarian failure, could nevertheless significantly deplete the size of the ovarian follicular pool at any particular age, hastening the time at which complete ovarian failure occurs.

Childhood and puberty (males)

Cyclophosphamide

Early studies suggested that the prepubertal testis was less sensitive to cytotoxics than the adult testis, but this assumption may no longer be justified. Cyclophosphamide produces the most severe damage, but this may be reversible over time. It is possible that the dose and duration of treatment with cyclophosphamide is a more important variable for sperm counts than the pubertal state. In a large follow-up study, 30 males who received cyclophosphamide between the ages of 3 and 17 (mean 9 years) for childhood nephrotic syndrome were assessed in adulthood for reproductive function: 60% were normospermic, 30% had reduced sperm counts and only 10% were azoospermic. There was an inverse correlation between sperm counts and both the duration of cyclophosphamide treatment and the total dose received. However, even the normospermic patients had raised FSH levels compared with controls, indicating some degree of compensated testicular damage (Watson, Rance & Bain, 1985). Another recent study showed that adult survivors of childhood cancer had smaller testicles than healthy controls and that this was a consequence of cyclophosphamide treatment. Testicular size was related to sperm production (Siimes & Rautonen, 1990). Another study assessed sperm parameters in men who had received childhood cyclophosphamide at a dose of 3 mg/kg body weight for 8 weeks. There was a decreased count, with an increase in the number of immotile and malformed sperm; the authors suggested that this was not sufficient to cause infertility (Trompeter, Evans & Barratt, 1981).

Chlorambucil

Chlorambucil, used before puberty in childhood nephrotic syndrome, has also been reported to have a marked affect on sperm count and testicular size. This led the authors to conclude that the quiescent state of the epithelium of the seminiferous tubules does not protect against chlorambucil toxicity (Guesry, Lenoir & Broyer, 1978).

Childhood and puberty (females)

Cyclophosphamide

The ovaries of prepubertal girls may be more resistant to the toxic gonadal effects of alkylating agents than those of adult women. However, primary ovarian failure can still occur and appears to be dose related. Three of twelve girls receiving combination chemotherapy for acute lymphatic leukaemia developed ovarian failure and all three had received cyclophosphamide. Treatment of prepubertal and pubertal girls with doses of cyclophosphamide of 525 mg/kg or less appears to be compatible with subsequent ovulatory cycles in the majority of patients (Damewood & Grochow, 1986). However the long-term effects in women have not yet been evaluated and it is possible that doses not associated with immediate ovarian failure may still provoke a premature menopause.

Lentz and colleagues assessed gonadal function in boys and girls treated with cyclophosphamide for nephrotic syndrome. In children receiving treatment before or during puberty, spermatic dysfunction was noted in 6 of 15 boys but there was no menstrual disturbance in any of the six girls. In postpubertal children, all four treated boys had sperm dysfunction but the seven treated girls had no evidence of an ovulatory disturbance at the time of follow-up (Lentz *et al.*,1977).

Single-agent chemotherapy

The alkylating agents have been the single agents most widely studied for their effects on reproductive function. There are, however a few reports of other drugs used in isolation having a detrimental influence on fertility.

Methotrexate

Adult men

Methotrexate is an antimetabolite that acts as a folinic acid antagonist and in general appears to have little effect on spermatogenesis. It has been proposed that there is a significant barrier to the passage of methotrexate across the blood-seminiferous tubule barrier, although reports have demonstrated severe reductions in sperm counts in certain individuals. This is probably related to the high dose used in these patients.

The drug acts on tissues with a high mitotic activity and, therefore, affects the rapidly dividing primitive sperm cells, notably the spermatogonia and spermatocytes. In some cases, the drug has been administered to non-cancer patients. One report describes a man treated with methotrexate for psoriasis, with a total dose of 800 mg. Serial analyses of seminal fluid demonstrated low sperm counts and a high number of morphologically abnormal forms. These disturbances resolved after the drug was discontinued. Recommencing therapy was associated with another reduction in count. Despite this, gonadotrophin levels remained normal (Sussman & Leonard, 1980). Another study looked at high-dose methotrexate in men being treated for osteosarcoma (Shamberger *et al.*, 1981). Approximately 50% developed severe oligozoospermia associated with raised FSH levels during or immediately after treatment. Sperm concentration and hormone levels both returned to normal after the completion of therapy.

Three cases of erectile dysfunction and inability to ejaculate have also been recorded in men receiving 12.5 mg methotrexate weekly for arthritis. Normal sexual function returned on discontinuing the drug though at the expense of worsening arthritis (Blackburn & Alarcón, 1989).

Adult women

In women, high-dose methotrexate appears to have no effect on ovarian function (Shamberger *et al.*, 1981). It is frequently used in the chemotherapy of choriocarcinoma. Rustin *et al.*, (1984) noted that 187 of 217 women who wished to become pregnant after methotrexate therapy had children. Interestingly, 37 of the women who did succeed in having a baby had also received cyclophosphamide.

Other single agents

Corticosteroids

Early studies suggested that prednisolone at a dose of 30 mg/day for 15 days causes reduced sperm counts and motility. This is associated with evidence of spermatogenic arrest at testicular biopsy (Mancini *et al.*, 1966). Full recovery had not occurred 6 months after the cessation of a 30 day trial. Sperm abnormalities have also been demonstrated in 10 men using topical cortisone for psoriasis (Grunnet, Nyfors & Hansen, 1977). The significance of these earlier reports, however, must be questionable. Higher dosage steroid regimens are now normal practice in the therapy of male infertility resulting from antisperm antibodies, and no detrimental effect on sperm parameters has been reported (Hendry *et al.*, 1990).

Mitotane

Mitotane has been used to treat adrenocortical carcinoma. One case report describes a patient who developed impotence as a result of testicular failure at the time of mitotane therapy. Testicular biopsy showed atrophy of seminiferous tubules but normal Leydig cells. Libido gradually improved and testosterone and gonadotrophin levels normalised over the next 4 years (Sparagana, 1987).

Vincristine

An assessment of 55 adult males who had been treated in childhood for various forms of malignancy showed that 28 (51%) were azoospermic. Although many different therapeutic regimens had been used, the authors showed by a multivariate statistical analysis that the use of vincristine had the most significant independent effect on the risk of azoospermia. The risk was five times greater than in patients who did not receive vincristine (Rautonen, Koskimies & Siimes, 1992).

Combination chemotherapy

Combinations of chemotherapeutic agents are commonly employed and often have significant deleterious effects on testicular and ovarian function. It is not usually possible to determine which agent in a pharmacological cocktail is responsible for the adverse effect observed, although regimens employing alkylating agents are an exception. The toxicity may be additive and even synergistic. Many therapeutic regimens are used and it is convenient to break them down into the disease states for which they are prescribed

Hodgkin's disease

Adult men

The MOPP (mustine, vincristine, procarbazine and prednisolone) regimen was first developed in 1964. It has proved efficacy in that 80% of men treated remained disease free after 10 years. This increased survival in a number of young patients has led to the desire for preservation of fertility in these men and women.

However two factors mitigate against this: the effect of the disease and the effect of chemotherapy treatment.

Effect of Hodgkin's disease on fertility. Hodgkin's disease affects sperm function. In a recent 7 year study, two thirds of 92 men with Hodgkin's disease had an abnormality of sperm count, motility or morphology before treatment, although gonadotrophin and testosterone levels were within the normal range (Viviani *et al.*, 1991). Another study looked at pretreatment sperm quality before cryopreservation in men with Hodgkin's disease. Compared with non-Hodgkin's controls, all sperm parameters were depressed. This included the sperm motility following thawing of the cryopreserved specimens. Of course this has considerable implications for the future fertility of young men with Hodgkin's disease (Redman *et al.*, 1987). In an assessment by Chapman *et al.*, (1981), 43% of men with Hodgkin's disease were described as subfertile on the basis of either impotence or 'inadequate' sperm counts prior to chemotherapy being initiated. Abnormalites of testicular histology were found in eight of nine pretreatment testicular biopsies.

Effect of chemotherapy for Hodgkin's disease on fertility. The second factor that mitigates against fertility in young men with Hodgkin's disease relates to the severe gonadal toxicity of the combination chemotherapy regimens. Many recent studies have assessed gonadal response to treatment comparing regimens such as MOPP, MVPP, COPP and ABVD (see Table 4.2). A prospective Italian study showed that MOPP produced azoospermia in 97% of patients whereas ABVD had a lesser effect, inducing oligozoospermia in 54%. Following treatment, FSH levels were elevated in the MOPP group and spermatogenesis only recovered in 3 of 21 patients. FSH levels were normal in the ABVD group and sperm function recovered in all cases (Viviani *et al.*, 1985). A retrospective study of these two regimens confirmed these findings (Anselmo *et al.*, 1990). It is presumed that the alkylating agent in MOPP (mustine) and procarbazine,

Table 4.2. *Some combination drug regimens used in chemotherapy*

Regimen	Drugs
MOPP	Mustine, vincristine (oncovin), procarbazine, prednisolone
MVPP	Mustine, vinblastine, procarbazine, prednisolone
COPP	Chlorambucil, vincristine, procarbazine, prednisolone
ABVD	Doxorubicin, bleomycin, vinblastine, dacarbazine

which has some alkylating activity, are responsible for the gonadal toxicity. Similar severe toxicity is associated with MVPP. Chapman *et al.,* (1981) reported that 100% of 14 men treated with MVPP developed azoospermia within 1 to 2 months of commencing therapy. This was associated with marked elevations in serum FSH levels. Possibly the use of alkylating agents in combination chemotherapy regimens may cause more long-lasting testicular damage than their use as single-agent therapy. This is related to additive damage at different sites. Mustine kills mature germ cells as well as destroying germinal epithelium, and vinblastine arrests primitive germ cells.

Male sexual dysfunction. Apart from the effect of chemotherapy on spermatogenesis, many men being treated for Hodgkin's disease develop sexual dysfunction. Half of the men in one study reported a decrease in libido at the time of diagnosis but this group increased to over 80% during therapy (Chapman *et al.,* 1981). This may be a consequence of the stress associated with the diagnosis of cancer, although only 10% of men were impotent before therapy commenced. Alternatively, the unpleasant systemic side effects of chemotherapy are likely to lead to a reduction in interest in sexual relations.

Adult women

In contrast to the situation in men, ovarian function does not appear to be adversely affected by Hodgkin's disease before treatment. The ovarian response to chemotherapy depends on the age of the patient and the type and dose of treatment.

In a long-term follow-up study of 28 women treated using the MVPP regimen, 22 became amenorrhoeic with associated oestrogen deficiency. In this group of patients, the ovarian damage was thought to be permanent, i.e. the patients had become menopausal (Waxman *et al.,* 1982).

Influence of duration of treatment. Normal ovarian function was retained in 24% of patients receiving six cycles of MVPP chemotherapy but only in 5% of patients who needed seven or more cycles. All patients who received 12 cycles of chemotherapy developed ovarian failure irrespective of age (Chapman, Sutcliffe & Malpas, 1979a). ·

Influence of age. Analysis of the effects of patient age and duration of therapy in one study showed that a third of 16 patients who were less than 29 years old developed ovarian failure in response to MVPP therapy for Hodgkin's disease. This increased to 84% in a group of 25 patients who were 30 years or older (Chapman, 1984).

Horning *et al.* (1981) calculated the probability of retaining regular menstruation in women in relationship to age and modality of treatment. The association of chemotherapy and total lymphoid irradiation was more likely to result in ovarian dysfunction than chemotherapy alone. Following chemotherapy alone, a 20-year-old woman had nearly an 80% chance of regular periods after treatment. However this decreased to only approximately 30% in a 30 year old. The obvious correlation of this is that the chances of pregnancy are severely reduced if menstruation is irregular or if the patient becomes amenorrhoeic.

It is probable that ovarian damage occurs even in women who do not become amenorrhoeic during therapy. This is manifested by an earlier menopause than would be anticipated naturally. This phenomenon is also age related so that ovarian failure occurred within 1 year of cessation of therapy in all patients over the age of 38 years, whereas in younger patients there was a gradual decrease in menstrual frequency over a period of several years (Schilsky *et al.*, 1981). Therefore, age, number of cycles of treatment and regularity of menstruation can all be used to try to predict the chances of future fertility in women being treated for Hodgkin's disease.

Ovarian failure obviously prevents the possibility of future conception, but there are more immediate effects that can also be distressing. These are the typical menopausal symptoms, the commonest of which is hot flushes. Many young women find these embarrassing. Low oestrogen levels are also associated with a reduction in vaginal lubrication during coitus and a thinning of the vaginal epithelium, both of which contribute to painful intercourse. It is not surprising that many women experience a profound change in their sexual relationships following ovarian failure induced by chemotherapy: 70% of women claimed to have little or no libido when followed for a mean time of 3 years after combined chemotherapy. It has been estimated that the rate of breakdown of couples in which the woman has developed ovarian failure between the ages of 25 to 30 is four times greater than in the general population (Chapman, Sutcliffe & Malpas, 1979b).

Children

Pubertal boys receiving MOPP chemotherapy for Hodgkin's disease had a high incidence of gynaecomastia and germinal aplasia (Sherins, Olweny & Ziegler, 1978). This developed at a mean time of 28 months after treatment and was associated with raised FSH and LH levels and reduced testosterone. This combination suggests damage to both the Leydig cells and the germinal epithelium. Presumably the damage to the Leydig cells causes a reduction in testosterone levels, which induces breast development.

One recent study examined testicular function in 28 adults who had been treated for Hodgkin's disease in childhood with chemotherapy (usually chlorambucil, vinblastine, procarbazine and prednisolone) with or without radiotherapy. Nearly all patients had elevated FSH levels (persisting up to 17 years after treatment in some cases) and 11 of 13 who had semen analyses performed were azoospermic (Shafford *et al.*, 1993). Another study showed a similar high rate of damage to the testicular function in men who had received COPP/MOPP combination therapy as prepubertal boys. All patients examined were azoospermic. The authors suggested that an ABVD protocol may be an alternative that would minimise testicular damage (Dhabhar *et al,*. 1993).

Testicular tumours

More than 95% of patients with testicular cancer can now be cured with appropriate chemotherapy (Fox & Loehrer, 1991). With such high cure rates, the reduction of toxicity is an important aim of current treatments. In this respect, there has been much progress since the mid-1980s. However, testicular tumours clearly affect fertility potential. A review of the literature shows that 20% of patients are azoospermic and 64% oligozoospermic before any treatment (Kreuser, Klingsmüller & Thiel, 1993).

Cisplatin

Cisplatin is a platinum analogue that interacts with sites on DNA, RNA or proteins to form covalent links similar to alkylation reactions, thereby preventing DNA transcription and synthesis.

In the past, drug treatment of testicular cancer was invariably thought to be associated with permanent infertility. The introduction of cisplatinum-based therapy challenged this traditional viewpoint. In a study in 1983, patients with non-seminomatous testicular cancers were treated with vinblastine and bleomycin and in some (24 of 29) cisplatin was a third agent (Lange *et al.*, 1983). Most of the patients also had retroperitoneal lymphadenectomy. This procedure caused disturbances of ejaculation, although in many patients this either resolved spontaneously or could be treated pharmacologically. The chemotherapy profoundly depressed sperm production during treatment. However in 75% of the patients, FSH levels had normalised and/or live sperm were present in the ejaculate when retesting was performed 18 months later.

A recent paper from Norway compared gonadal function in males following either infradiaphragmatic radiotherapy or three to four cycles of cisplatin-based chemotherapy (Aass *et al.*, 1991). Multiple sperm parameters were assessed at a median interval of 3 years after the discontinuation of treatment. Both therapies significantly elevated serum FSH levels but had no effect on serum testosterone. Standard chemotherapy caused less reduction in sperm count than radiotherapy, but recovery of gonadal function was delayed after more intensive chemotherapy. Patient age and gonadal function before treatment correlated well with long-term gonadal toxicity. It was encouraging that in those patients who had normal gonadal function before treatment, the risk of permanent treatment-induced infertility was minimal following the standard cisplatin-based regimen.

More significant toxicity was noted in a German study of patients with disseminated testicular cancer treated with a combination of cisplatin, vinblastine and bleomycin and/or adriamycin (Kreuser *et al.*, 1986). Hormone levels were measured and semen analyses performed before, during and following (maximum follow-up, 6 years) chemotherapy. There were no changes in LH, testosterone or prolactin levels, but 20% of patients had increased FSH prior to treatment because of testicular dysfunction. All patients developed azoospermia associated with significantly elevated FSH levels. However, 80% of the patients assessed in the third year after chemotherapy showed normalisation of FSH and all had recovery of spermatogenesis. There was, however, an abnormally high number of immotile sperm and only a minority of men were able to father children.

A similar, albeit retrospective, assessment was performed in another study of men treated with the same combination chemotherapy (Johnson *et al.*, 1984). This group were studied in the first year after completing chemotherapy. All showed elevated FSH, but in contrast to the German study, LH concentrations were also raised. Testosterone was nearly always normal. In two thirds of the patients, FSH and LH levels recovered to normal or nearly normal after 24 months. Semen samples provided within 2 years of therapy were azoospermic in 71% of men but this fell to 17% in men who produced their sperm after more than 2 years from the end of therapy. The authors concluded that this regimen caused destruction of the germinal epithelium as well as transient Leydig cell dysfunction, although this did not coexist with clinical hypogonadism. This study also demonstrated that chemotherapy for testicular cancer had a severe but usually transient effect on sperm production and that recovery or at least partial recovery of fertility was possible in the majority of treated men.

The effect of cisplatin-based therapy is probably dose dependent. A study of patients treated with cisplatin, etoposide and bleomycin for testicular tumours showed that 19% of those receiving conventional doses of cisplatin (20 mg/m^2) developed azoospermia. In contrast, 47% of those on high-dose cisplatin (40 mg/m^2) became azoospermic. The serum FSH concentration was greater in the high-dose group (Petersen *et al.*, 1994).

Protection against gonadal toxicity

Gonadotrophin-releasing hormone analogues

GnRH analogues act by causing down-regulation of pituitary GnRH receptors. This leads to suppression of pituitary FSH and LH production and consequently to hypogonadism. In a mouse model, GnRH administered to males before cyclophosphamide protected against disruption of spermatogenesis (Glode, Robinson & Gould, 1981). Presumably, the rate of spermatogenesis is suppressed and, therefore, it is less sensitive to chemotherapeutic damage. Unfortunately the results in human studies have been less impressive. Six men with lymphoma received GnRH analogue therapy before and during chemotherapy. Despite clinical hypogonadism and oligozoospermia or azoospermia, all patients developed testicular failure following treatment (Johnson *et al.*, 1985).

A group of 30 men and 18 women with Hodgkin's disease were randomly allocated to receive GnRH analogue therapy before and during chemotherapy. At follow-up, for up to 3 years, all the GnRH analogue-treated men and all the controls who did not receive analogue were profoundly oligozoospermic. Approximately half of the women in each group were amenorrhoeic, showing that GnRH analogue offered no protection despite being given at doses that induced hypogonadism (Waxman *et al.*, 1987).

A recent literature review reported on three studies comparing gonadal damage in patients receiving chemotherapy with and without GnRH analogues. No differences were found between treated and untreated patients. The authors concluded that the evidence for lack of gonadal protection by GnRH analogues was sufficiently convincing that further clinical trials were unwarranted (Kreuser *et al.*, 1993).

Combined contraceptive pill

Before GnRH analogues were widely available, initial reports had suggested that ovarian function might be protected by using the combined contraceptive pill. However, this was not born out by more extensive studies and it appears as if there are no effective pharmacological means to protect either the male or female gonad from chemotherapy-induced damage (Gradishar & Schilsky, 1988; Kreser *et al.*, 1993).

Cryostorage of sperm

An alternative strategy to protect reproductive function is to store the gametes before chemotherapy commences. This has been widely adopted for the cryopreservation of sperm and if time allows most young men should be offered this facility before treatment. However this certainly does not guarantee the future ability to father children.

There are three main problems associated with sperm cryostorage in cancer patients. Freezing and subsequent thawing kills large numbers of healthy motile sperm. For example, many sperm banks reject over 50% of healthy young men who wish to offer their sperm for donation because the sperm that survive the freezing process are of inadequate quality to achieve fertilisation. In addition, many men with cancer have abnormal sperm parameters as a consequence of their disease and the sperm is of low fertility potential even before freezing. A further and very significant problem relates to the patient's emotional state. Having been informed that he suffers from cancer and that he needs to have a course of toxic chemotherapy that will probably destroy the possibility of fathering children naturally, he is then asked to produce several specimens of sperm by masturbation. Some men find this unacceptable, others impossible.

There have been some recent developments in assisted conception technology that may be of great benefit to men with cryopreserved sperm. It is often suggested that *in vitro* fertilisation using the cryopreserved sperm should be used when the couple wish to conceive. It is now possible to microinject individual sperm directly inside the egg and achieve high rates of fertilisation and pregnancy (Van Steirteghem *et al.*, 1993). This technique, called intracytoplasmic sperm injection, or ICSI, is highly suitable for sperm of even extremely poor quality and offers a major breakthrough to patients who only have frozen sperm available.

Currently the techniques of gamete cryostorage do not extend to human eggs and so this possibility is not available to women undergoing cancer chemotherapy. The human egg is a very large cell and because of this is highly susceptible to damage by freezing. Nevertheless, there is much research work being performed in this area and there have been reports of human pregnancy following egg freezing (Chen, 1986). It is, therefore likely that human egg storage will be available by the end of the 1990s.

Hormone-replacement therapy

Currently it is not possible to preserve fertility in women having certain forms of chemotherapy. However, treatment is available for other forms of sexual dysfunction provoked by cancer chemotherapy. A premature menopause may result from chemotherapeutic-induced damage to eggs and ovarian follicles. This can have serious effects on morbidity. After the menopause for example, womens' likelihood of developing coronary artery disease increases to equal that of men. Oestrogen protection of bones is lost, leading to osteoporosis, which can result in fractures of the vertebral spine and the neck of the femur. Oestrogen deficiency also affects sexuality both physically by reducing vaginal secretions and psychologically by a decrease in libido. For all these reasons hormone-replacement therapy (HRT) should be offered to all women with drug-induced oestrogen deficiency provided that the original cancer was not oestrogen dependent.

Teratogenicity of chemotherapy

A final aspect of reproduction following cancer chemotherapy of great importance to patients is the risks of abnormality in their future offspring as a consequence of genetic mutations induced by their treatment. The clinical studies that have been performed here are fortunately reassuring. Damewood and Grochow (1986) reviewed the evidence from a group of studies analysing pregnancy outcome in 468 conceptions in patients treated by chemotherapy and/or radiotherapy. There was no greater risk of

68   Cancer chemotherapy

miscarriage or fetal abnormality than in the general population. However, it has not yet been possible to assess the risks to the gene pool of subsequent generations.

References

Aass, N., Fossa, S. D., Theodorsen, L. & Norman, N. (1991). Prediction of long-term gonadal toxicity after standard treatment for testicular cancer. *European Journal of Cancer*, 27, 1087–91.

Anselmo, A. P., Cartoni, C., Bellantuono, P., Maurizi-Enrici, R., Aboulkair, N. & Ermini, M. (1990). Risk of infertility in patients with Hodgkin's disease treated with ABVD vs MOPP vs ABVD/MOPP. *Haematologica*, 75, 155–8.

Blackburn, W. D. & Alarcón, G. S. (1989). Impotence in three rheumatoid arthritis patients treated with methotrexate. *Arthritis and Rheumatism*, 32, 1341–2.

Chapman, R. M. (1983) Gonadal injury resulting from chemotherapy. *American Journal of Industrial Medicine*, 4, 149–61.

Chapman, R. M. (1984). Effect of cytotoxic therapy on sexuality and gonadal function. In *Toxicity of Chemotherapy*, ed. M. C. Perry & J. W. Yarbo, pp. 343–63. Orlando; Grune & Stratton.

Chapman, R. M., Sutcliffe, S. B. & Malpas, J. S. (1979a). Cytotoxic induced ovarian failure in women with Hodgkin's disease. I. Hormone function. *Journal of the American Medical Association*, 242, 1877–81.

Chapman, R. M., Sutcliffe, S. B. & Malpas, J. S. (1979b). Cytotoxic induced ovarian failure in women with Hodgkin's disease. II. Effects on sexual function. *Journal of the American Medical Association*, 242, 1882–4.

Chapman, R. M., Sutcliffe, S. B. & Malpas, J. S. (1981). Male gonadal dysfunction in Hodgkins disease. A prospective study. *Journal of the American Medical Association*, 245, 1323–8.

Chen, C. (1986). Pregnancy after human oocyte cryopreservation. *Lancet*, i, 884–6.

Damewood, M.D. & Grochow, L. B. (1986). Prospects for fertility after chemotherapy or radiation for neoplastic disease. *Fertility and Sterility*, 45, 443–59.

Dhabhar, B. N., Malhotra, H., Joseph, R., Garde, S., Bhasin, S, Sheth, A. & Advani, S. H. (1993). Gonadal function in prepubertal boys following treatment for Hodgkin's disease. *American Journal of Pediatric Hematology/Oncology*, 15, 306–10.

Etteldorf, J. N., West, C. D., Pitcock, J. K. & Williams, D. L. (1976). Gonadal function, testicular histology, and meiosis following cyclophosphamide therapy in patients with nephrotic syndrome. *Journal of Pediatrics*, 88, 206–12.

Fairley, K. F., Barrie, J. U. & Johnson W. (1972). Sterility and testicular atrophy related to cyclophosphamide therapy. *Lancet*, i, 1212–14.

Fox, E. P. & Loehrer, P. J. Sr (1991). Chemotherapy for advanced testicular cancer. *Hematology/Oncology Clinics of North America*, 5, 1173–87.

Glode, L. M., Robinson, J. & Gould, S. F. (1981). Protection from cyclophosphamide-induced testicular damage with an analogue of gonadotropin-releasing hormone. *Lancet*, 1, 1132–4.

Gradishar, W. L. & Schilsky, R. L. (1988). Effects of cancer treatment on the reproductive system. *Critical Reviews in Oncology/Hematology*, 8, 153–71.

Grunnet, E., Nyfors, A. & Hansen K.B. (1977). Studies on human semen in topical corticosteroid treated and in methotrexate treated patients. *Dermatologica*, 154, 78–84.

Guesry, P., Lenoir, G. & Broyer, M. (1978). Gonadal effects of chlorambucil given to prepubertal and pubertal boys for nephrotic syndrome. *Journal of Pediatrics*, 92, 299–303.

Hendry, W. F., Hughes, L., Scammel, G., Pryor, J. & Hargreave T. B. (1990). *Lancet*, 335, 85–8.

Horning, S. J., Hoppe, R. T., Kaplan, H. S. & Rosenberg, S. A. (1981). Female reproductive potential after treatment for Hodgkin's disease. *New England Journal of Medicine*, 304, 1377–82.

Johansson, J. E., Andersson, S. O., Beckman, K. W., Lingardh, G. and Zador, G. (1987). Clinical evaluation of flutamide and estramustine as initial treatment of metastatic carcinoma of prostate. *Urology*, 29, 55–9.

Johnson, D. H., Hainsworth, J. D., Linde, R. B. & Greco, F. A. (1984). Testicular function following combination chemotherapy with cisplatin, vinblastine, and bleomycin. *Medical and Pediatric Oncology*, 12, 233–8.

Johnson, D. H., Linde, R., Hainsworth, J. D., Vale,W., Rivier, J., Stein, R., Flexner, J., van Welch, R. & Greco, F. A. (1985). Effect of a luteinizing hormone releasing hormone agonist given during combination chemotherapy on post-therapy fertility in male patients with lymphoma. *Blood*, 65, 832–6.

Kreuser, E. D., Harsch, U., Hetzel, W. D. & Schreml, W. (1986). Chronic gonadal toxicity in patients with testicular cancer after chemotherapy. *European Journal of Cancer and Clinical Oncology*, 22, 289–94.

Kreuser, E. D., Klingsmüller, D. & Thiel, E. (1993). The role of LHRH-analogues in protecting gonadal functions during chemotherapy and irradiation. *European Urology*, 23, 157–64.

Lange, P. H., Narayan, P., Vogelzang, N. J., Shafer, R. B., Kennedy, B. J. & Fraley, E. E. (1983). Return of fertility after treatment for nonseminomatous testicular cancer: changing concepts. *Journal of Urology*, 129, 1131–5.

Lentz, R. D., Bergstein, J., Steffes, M. W., Brown, D. R., Prem, K., Michael, A. F. & Vernier, R. L. (1977). Postpubertal evaluation of gonadal function following cyclophosphamide therapy before and during puberty. *Journal of Pediatrics*, 91, 385–94.

Mancini, R. E., Lavieri, J. C., Muller, F., Andrada, J. A. & Saraceni, D. J. (1966). Effect of prednisolone upon normal and pathologic human spermatogenesis. *Fertility and Sterility*, 17, 500–13.

Marmor, D., Grob Menendez, F., Duyck, F. & Delafontaine, D. (1992). Very late return of spermatogenesis after chlorambucil therapy: case reports. *Fertility and Sterility*, 58, 845–6.

Meistrich, M. L., Wilson, G., Brown, B. W., da Cunha, M. F. & Lipshultz, L. I. (1992). Impact of cyclophosphamide on long-term reduction in sperm count in men treated with combination chemotherapy for Ewing and soft tissue sarcomas. *Cancer*, 70, 2703–12.

Petersen, P. M., Hansen, S. W., Giwercman, A., Rorth, M. & Skakkebaek, N. E. (1994). Dose-dependent impairment of testicular function in patients treated with cisplatin-based chemotherapy for germ cell cancer. *Annals of Oncology*, 5, 355–8.

Rautonen, J., Koskimies, A. I. & Siimes, M. A. (1992). Vincristine is associated with the risk of azoospermia in adult male survivors of childhood malignancies. *European Journal of Cancer*, 28A, 1837–41.

Redman, J. R., Bajorunas, D. R., Goldstein, M. C., Evenson, D. P., Gralla, R. J., Lacher, M. J., Koziner, B., Lee, B. J., Straus, D. J., Clarkson, B. D., Feldschuh, R. & Feldschuh, J. (1987). Semen cryopreservation and artificial insemination for Hodgkin's disease. *Journal of Clinical Oncology*, 5, 233–8.

Rustin, G. J. S., Booth, M., Dent, J., Salt, S., Rustin, F. & Bagshawe, K. D. (1984). Pregnancy after cytotoxic chemotherapy for gestational trophoblastic tumours. *British Medical Journal*, 288, 103–6.

Schilsky, R. L., Lewis, B. J., Sherins, R. J & Young, R. C. (1980). Gonadal dysfunction in patients receiving chemotherapy for cancer. *Annals of Internal Medicine*, 93, 109–14.

Schilsky, R. L., Sherins, R. J., Hubbard, S. M., Wesley, M. N., Young, R. C. & DeVita, V. T. (1981). Long-term follow up of ovarian function in women treated with MOPP chemotherapy for Hodgkins disease. *American Journal of Medicine*, 71, 552–6.

Shafford, E. A., Kingston, J. E., Malpas, J. S., Plowman, P. N., Pritchard, J., Savage, M. O. & Eden, O. B. (1993). Testicular function following the treatment of Hodgkin's disease in childhood. *British Journal of Cancer*, 68, 1199–204.

Shalet, S. M. (1980). Effects of cancer chemotherapy on gonadal function of patients. *Cancer Treatment Reviews*, 7, 141–52.

Shamberger, R. C., Rosenberg, S. A., Seipp, C. A. & Sherins, R. J. (1981). Effects of high-dose methotrexate and vincristine on ovarian and testicular functions in patients undergoing postoperative adjuvant treatment of osteosarcoma. *Cancer Treatment Reports*, 65, 739–46.

Sherins, R. J., Olweny, C. L. M. & Ziegler, J. L. (1978). Gynecomastia and gonadal dysfunction in adolescent boys treated with combination chemotherapy for Hodgkin's disease. *New England Journal of Medicine*, 299, 12–16.

Siimes, M. A. & Rautonen, J. (1990). Small testicles with impaired production of sperm in adult male survivors of childhood malignancies. *Cancer*, 65, 1303–6.

Sparagana, M. (1987). Primary hypogonadism associated with o, p' DDD (mitotane) therapy. *Journal of Toxicology, Clinical Toxicology*, 25, 463–72.

Spitz, S. (1948). The histological effects of nitrogen mustards on human tumors and tissues. *Cancer*, 1, 383–98.

Sussman, A. & Leonard, J. M. (1980). Psoriasis, methotrexate, and oligospermia. *Archives of Dermatology*, 116, 215–17.

Trompeter, R. S., Evans, P. R. & Barratt, T. M. (1981). Gonadal function in boys with steroid-responsive nephrotic syndrome treated with cyclophosphamide for short periods. *Lancet*, i, 1177–9.

Van Steirteghem, A. C., Nagy, Z., Joris, H., Liu, J., Staessen, C., Smitz, J. & Devroey, P. (1993). High fertilisation and implantation rates after intracytoplasmic sperm injection. *Human Reproduction*, 8, 1061–6.

Viviani, S., Ragni, G., Santoro, A., Perotti, L., Caccamo, E., Negretti, E, Valagussa, P. & Bonadonna, G. (1991). Testicular dysfunction in Hodgkin's disease before and after treatment. *European Journal of Cancer*, 27, 1389–92.

Viviani, S., Santoro, A., Ragni, G., Bonfante, V., Bestetti, O. & Bonadonna, G. (1985). Gonadal toxicity after combination chemotherapy for Hodgkin's disease. Comparative results of MOPP vs ABVD. *European Journal of Cancer and Clinical Oncology*, 21, 601–5.

Warne, G. L., Fairley, K. F., Hobbs, J. B. & Martin F. I. R. (1973) Cyclophosphamide induced ovarian failure. *New England Journal of Medicine*, 289, 1159–62.

Watson, A. R., Rance, C. P. & Bain, J. (1985). Long term effects of cyclophosphamide on testicular function. *British Medical Journal*, 291, 1457–60.

Waxman, J. H., Ahmed, R., Smith, D., Wrigley, P.F., Gregory, W., Shalet, S., Crowther, T., Rees, L. H., Besser, G. M. Malpas, J. S. & Lister, T. A. (1987). Failure to preserve fertility in patients with Hodgkin's disease. *Cancer Chemotherapy and Pharmacology*, 19, 159–62.

Waxman, J. H., Terry, Y. A., Wrigley, P. F., Malpas, J. S., Rees, L. H., Besser, G. M. & Lister, T. A. (1982) Gonadal function in Hodgkin's disease: long term follow up of chemotherapy. *British Medical Journal*, 285, 1612–13.

5

Hormone therapy

Sex hormones

Oestrogens

Combined oral contraceptive pill

In 1993, a National Opinion Poll was carried out on behalf of a pharmaceutical company that manufactures contraceptive pills. This poll surveyed 1000 women in the 16 to 44 year age range. The combined oral contraceptive pill (OCP) was the most popular form of contraception used: 90% of women had used it at some time in their sexual history and 33% of women were current users.

The pill is designed to produce reversible infertility. The oestrogen component inhibits ovulation and the progestogen both balances the oestrogen (oestrogen unopposed by progestogen can induce endometrial cancer) and has contraceptive properties. As the therapeutic effect of the pill is to produce infertility, it is not relevant to discuss this aspect further. However, there have been a few reports linking OCP use to reduced libido. In a 1976 review of psychological effects of pill use, Kane reported that between 10 and 40% of users of OCPs suffered mild to moderate depressive syndromes, many also experiencing loss of libido (Kane, 1976). This figure does seem very high but these studies, which were all performed in the late 1960s and early 1970s, were concerned with hormone formulations that used much higher doses of oestrogen and different progestogens from those in current use. However, even a recent placebo-controlled study using modern triphasic contraception has shown that women using these pills reported significantly decreased sexual interest during the menstrual and post-menstrual phases of the cycle. This effect was unrelated to any influence of the pill on mood (Graham & Sherwin, 1993). In contrast, there is anecdotal evidence that women taking OCPs experience an increase in sexual desire as their concern about falling pregnant is alleviated.

Diethylstilboestrol

Diethylstilboestrol (DES) is a synthetic oestrogen with a chequered history. Between 1940 and 1970 it was given to approximately 2 to 4 million women in the USA and probably 10 000 women in the UK. DES was given prophylactically in threatened and recurrent abortion. It was also thought to be beneficial in the prophylaxis of pre-eclampsia (toxaemia of pregnancy), prematurity and perinatal mortality, although subsequent results showed this not to be the case. As a consequence of DES exposure, the female and even the male offspring of these women have a high incidence of reproductive tract malformations affecting both fertility and reproductive function. In addition, female offspring have 100 to 1000 times greater incidence of vaginal and cervical clear cell adenocarcinomas than normal. Pregnancy outcome is also adversely affected in daughters of exposed women, with an increased risk of premature labour, low birth weight and antepartum haemorrhage (Anon, 1991; Emens, 1994).

Fertility problems in DES-exposed daughters

In 1951–2, a double-blind controlled study of DES use in pregnancy was commenced at the Chicago Lying-in hospital. A group of 840 pregnant women were given DES and a second group of 806 women were given placebo. This study has allowed accurate long-term follow-up of the daughters of both DES-treated women and their controls, and 408 DES-exposed daughters and 388 unexposed daughters have been contacted for ongoing study. The long-term influence on fertility was reviewed by Senekjian et al., (1988). Of the total population, 207 exposed and 203 unexposed women had been trying to conceive. Primary infertility was reported by 33% of the exposed and 14% of non-exposed daughters. As might be expected, the infertility in the exposed daughters was more likely to result from a cervical, uterine or tubal factor than in the non-exposed women. None of the infertile control women had abnormalities of the uterine cavity, whereas abnormalities were present in 46% of the DES-exposed group. These abnormalities included T shaped or hypoplastic cavities, septate uteri, intrauterine adhesions and irregular uterine margins. Interestingly, tubal defects compatible with pelvic inflammatory disease appeared more common in DES-exposed daughters, although the reasons for this are unclear.

Other studies have shown an increased incidence of ovulation defects and second trimester abortion in DES-exposed women. There is conflicting evidence about whether the incidence of endometriosis is increased.

Ectopic pregnancies occur in 10 to 14% of DES daughters, presumably secondary to uterine or tubal abnormalities.

Fertility problems in DES-exposed sons

An equal number of male fetuses were exposed to DES during intrauterine life as exposed females. While most of the concern about DES exposure has centred on female offspring, a few studies have investigated males. Reproductive tract abnormalities and sperm defects occur in male offspring. A follow-up study of sons from the Chicago Lying-In hospital's original double-blind study showed anatomical abnormalities in 25% of DES-exposed males compared with 7% in control males. The most common abnormalities were epididymal cysts, small testes and small penises (Bibbo *et al.*, 1977).

Severe pathological changes were noted in the semen analyses of 18% of DES-exposed males but only in 8% of control subjects, although in this study few men had attempted conception so fertility could not be determined (Gill *et al.*, 1979).

Another study reported reduced sperm concentration in DES-exposed offspring compared with a non-exposed group (66.4 million/ml versus 101.4 million/ml). Furthermore in this study, zona-free hamster egg penetration tests, in which human sperm are used to inseminate hamster eggs, were performed. This is a reasonable model of the interaction between human sperm and human eggs. They found that DES-exposed males had poorer results than controls, suggesting reduced fertility (Stenchever *et al.*, 1981).

Progestogens

Until recently, natural progesterone could not be administered orally as it was broken down in the gastrointestinal tract. Micronised progesterone preparations are now available in some countries but synthetic progestogens are the most widely used. They are divided into two groups. The testosterone analogues include *norethisterone, norgestrel* and the norgestrel derivatives, i.e. *desogestrel, norgestimate* and *gestodene*. Progesterone derivatives are *allyloestrenol, dydrogesterone, hydroxyprogesterone* and *medroxyprogesterone*. Progestational agents have many uses in gynaecology. They are prescribed for contraception, menorrhagia, dysmenorrhoea, premenstrual syndrome, endometriosis, threatened miscarriage and adjuvant therapy for endometrial carcinoma. Progestogens are also added to oestrogens in hormone-replacement therapy in women being treated for perimenopausal symptoms.

The effects on reproductive function depend on several factors including the molecular structure, i.e. whether the drug is a progesterone or testosterone derivative, the dose and the duration of administration.

Progestogen-only contraception

Progestogen-only contraception is often prescribed to women in circumstances where oestrogen-containing oral contraceptives are contraindicated. This group includes older women, smokers, breast-feeding mothers, etc. The drug is taken at the same time each day throughout the month and exerts a contraceptive action at several sites. The cervical mucus becomes thick and resistant to the passage of sperm, the endometrium is rendered unfavourable for embryonic implantation, smooth muscle motility in the fallopian tube is reduced and, in approximately 50% of women, ovulation is suppressed.

Progestogens may be administered by other routes as long-acting contraceptives. Intramuscular injections have been available for several years but recent developments include progesterone-containing vaginal rings, intrauterine coils and subcuticular implants. There is evidence from one study that women discontinuing the intramuscular depot progestogen medroxyprogesterone acetate (Depo-provera) take longer to conceive than women stopping the combined contraceptive pill and those discontinuing conventional intrauterine contraceptive devices (Pardthaisong, 1984). Two years after cessation of contraceptive measures, there was a significantly lower cumulative conception rate in Depo-provera users than in combined contraceptive pill users. This probably results from a residual effect of the drug in some women.

Progestogens in other indications

Progestogens are frequently prescribed for the management of abnormal menstrual bleeding. In this indication, they are usually prescribed cyclically, e.g. in the last 2 weeks of the menstrual cycle. With this duration of administration, they do not interfere with ovulation and, therefore, do not significantly interfere with fertility. However loss of libido is a recognised side effect.

In the treatment of endometriosis, progestogens may be prescribed continuously for 3 months or more. This period of administration usually provokes amenorrhoea secondary to suppression of ovulation, and transient infertility will result.

In men, progestogens have also been investigated for treatment of benign prostatic hypertrophy. The use of an injectable preparation, gestonorone, administered once a week for 2 to 3 months led to subjective and objective evidence of improvement of prostatic symptoms but was associated with impotence in two thirds of the 30 men treated (Palanca & Juco, 1977).

Androgens

Testosterone and male contraception

A World Health Organization task force reported in 1990 on the treatment of 271 fertile men with 200 mg testosterone enanthate by weekly intramuscular injection as a contraceptive method (World Health Organisation, 1990). Two thirds became azoospermic within a mean time of 120 days. Once azoospermia had persisted for 1 year, the mean time to recovery of sperm concentration to pretreatment levels, after discontinuation of injections, was 6.7 months. Only one pregnancy occurred in 1486 months of treatment (0.8 per 100 person years). Decreases in FSH, LH and testicular volume were noted, but values returned to normal in the recovery phase. The contraceptive efficacy was better than for the female OCP. Three men withdrew from the study because of increased aggressiveness and libido. Possible future developments include depot testosterone preparations with longer dosing intervals of several months. In order to improve the percentage of men rendered azoospermic by testosterone, other agents have been added to the regimen. These include progestogens, GnRH agonists and recently GnRH antagonists. However, none of these regimens to date has improved upon the azoospermia rate achieved with testosterone alone.

Anabolic steroid abuse

There is an increasing trend by sportsmen and women to self administer anabolic steroids (AS). They are used to develop muscle bulk, strength and enhance physique. This is of particular interest to body builders, weight lifters, sprinters and other power athletes (Marshall, 1988). A recent review examined the significant health risks associated with pharmacological doses of androgens (Friedl, 1990) . These include altered lipid profiles increasing the risk of coronary artery disease, increased oestrogenisation leading to strokes, and cholestatic jaundice. Peliosis hepatitis, a very rare hepatic disease consisting of blood cysts in the liver, also occurs. Androgen-associated hepatocellular tumours have also been described. Many of these health risks are particularly associated with the orally active 17-alkylated androgens, e.g. oxandrolone, oxymetholone, methandrostenolone and stanozolol. The injectable esters testosterone enathate and nandrolone decanoate may carry less health risks but introduce the problem of needle sharing leading to sepsis, hepatitis and HIV infection. Much of the health risk information has been derived from studies of patients receiving therapeutic doses of androgens under medical supervision. The potential magnitude of risk associated with AS abuse is only just becoming apparent.

It is only recently that investigations have begun to assess the sexual function of athletes abusing AS. As early as 1938, a marked increase in erectile capacity and sex drive was noted in men being treated with testosterone propionate for impotence. In 1943, anabolic steroids were used in 101 women with a variety of endocrine disorders. Libido increased in 90%. In 20% it was noted that the stimulation was excessive (Uzych, 1992).

It is now apparent that the pattern of AS use in athletes differs greatly from that used in therapeutic regimens. Pope and co-workers recently sent a questionnaire to 41 athletes drawn from 38 gymnasia on the East and West Coast of the USA. Steroids were typically taken in cycles of 4 to 12 weeks. Athletes had between 1 and 30 cycles of AS. Often several drugs are taken simultaneously (stacking) including the self administration of veterinary preparations. It was difficult to estimate the actual dose equivalency of many of the preparations to therapeutic drugs, but it was estimated that many subjects took between 10 and 100 times the doses reported in medical studies (Pope & Katz, 1988).

Anecdotal reports have suggested that athletes on low-dose androgenic anabolic steroids experience reduction in libido and even impotence (van der Zon, 1990). A recent controlled study looked at sexual performance objectively and compared this with the subjective impressions of sexual function in athletes who were current users of AS. This was then compared with past users and non-users of AS (Moss, Panzak & Tarter, 1993). This study was revealing because it helps to resolve some of the inconsistencies of previous reports. Current users of AS reported significantly more episodes of sexual activity leading to orgasm than did past users or non-users. There was no difference between the three groups in the qualitative enjoyment of sexual activity but current and past users *believed* that AS enhanced sexual function.

However, 20% of current users reported difficulty maintaining erections during sexual activity. This was not reported by any past or non-users. This result helps to explain why previous studies have shown some men experiencing increased libido whereas others reported a decrease. Sexual appetite is androgen dependent but erectile function is not. Therefore, although the current AS users in this study had increased sexual thoughts, their bodies were not always able to keep pace with their desires.

Danazol

Danazol, a derivative of 17 α-ethinyltestosterone, has both progestogenic and androgenic actions. It is used mainly for the treatment of endometriosis but is also prescribed in mastalgia and menorrhagia. In endometriosis, it is administered continuously for up to 9 months. At high doses, danazol suppresses ovulation and produces infertility. At lower doses, ovulation can still occur and patients should be advised to use non-hormonal contraceptive precautions as danazol can lead to virilisation of female fetuses. Loss of libido is an occasionally reported side effect in some studies. In a large study of over 200 patients treated with 400 or 800 mg danazol per day, only three patients withdrew from treatment for this reason, although they all had other side effects as well (Buttram, Reiter & Ward, 1985). A non-randomised study compared the side effect profile of danazol and *gestrinone* (an antigonadotrophin with androgenic and progestogenic properties similar to danazol). Both compounds were associated with a similar incidence of reduced libido of approximately 10% (Candiani *et al.*, 1990). However, a recent large European multicentre study compared danazol at a starting dose of 600 mg/day with a GnRH agonist and specifically recorded the patients' assessments of their libido before treatment and again every 4 weeks during treatment for 6 months. In this study, a reduction in libido was recorded in 52% of 103 patients on danazol (Shaw, 1992). This was a much higher incidence than in the other studies cited but probably illustrates the point that if sexual information is to be elicited from patients it must be specifically requested.

Antihormones

Agonists of GnRH

Agonists of GnRH are a recently introduced novel class of compound with many applications in gynaecology and the treatment of hormone-dependent tumours. They act by binding to pituitary receptors at the site where naturally occurring GnRH would normally attach. Initially they mimic the effect of GnRH and stimulate the production of FSH and LH by the pituitary. However, pituitary stores of FSH and LH become exhausted and are not replaced. Low pituitary FSH and LH levels result in lack of stimulation of the ovaries in women and the testicles in men, resulting in hypogonadism. This situation persists for as long as the agonist is administered. These drugs, therefore, induce a reversible medical castration. GnRH agonists can be administered in the form of a nasal spray, subcutaneous injections or monthly intramuscular depot preparations. All GnRH agonists have a similar side effect profile. Currently available preparations include *buserelin*, *naferelin*, *goserelin* and *leuprolide*. In women, GnRH agonists are frequently used for the treatment of endometriosis. In this condition, they are administered for a maximum of 6 months. Women having surgery for fibroids sometimes receive 3 months preoperative treatment with a GnRH agonist to reduce the volume of the fibroid before surgery. The use of GnRH agonists has also been proposed in menorrhagia, premenstrual syndrome and adjuvant therapy in breast cancer. In men, they are usually prescribed for adjuvant treatment of prostatic carcinoma and have also been assessed in the treatment of hypersexuality disorders and for male contraception.

The side effect profile of GnRH agonists can easily be deduced from knowledge of their mechanism of action. Women are rendered effectively menopausal during treatment. They are infertile as ovulation is suppressed. Furthermore, low circulating oestrogen levels are associated with vaginal dryness (a frequent cause of pain during sexual intercourse) and lack of libido (Shaw, 1988). In the European study cited above in which women with endometriosis were treated with danazol or a GnRH agonist, 66% of the 204 patients randomised to GnRH agonist noted a reduction in libido (Shaw, 1992). Fortunately these effects are rapidly reversible following cessation of treatment. These compounds should not be administered to women for longer than 6 months as the prolonged hypo-oestrogenic state leads to a measurable reduction in bone density that may be irreversible.

Men being treated with GnRH agonists for prostatic cancer also experience loss of libido (Koutsilieris *et al.*, 1986). A recent study of leuprolide in the treatment of benign prostatic hyperplasia confirmed that erectile function and sexual activity was lost during therapy (Eri & Tveter, 1994). This effect has been put to clinical use in the treatment of men with deviant sexual behaviour (Thibaut, Cordier & Kuhn, 1993).

Antiandrogens

Cyproterone acetate and spironolactone

Cyproterone acetate (CPA) is an antiandrogen with strong progestogenic activity. It acts by reducing circulating testosterone concentrations but also inhibits the action of natural occurring testosterone and its metabolic products at the receptor site.

Spironolactone is an aldosterone antagonist that has been used to treat primary aldosteronism, hypertension and hypokalaemia. Its use in these conditions is limited by the adverse side effects, including decreased libido, impotence and gynaecomastia in men and menstrual disturbance in women. This side effect profile led to its therapeutic use to treat hirsutism. Spironolactone causes variable suppression of glandular testosterone secretion and also competes with androgens at the target cell level.

Antiandrogens have several therapeutic uses in circumstances where the disorder is related to overproduction of androgens or raised androgen activity in the skin. The most common uses are for the treatment of hirsutism, seborrhoea and acne in women. They have also been employed in the treatment of androgenic alopecia and hypersexuality in women and precocious puberty in children. CPA has been prescribed for male sexual offenders.

As androgens are implicated in human sexuality, certainly in males and probably in females, it might be expected that the use of antiandrogens would impact negatively on sexual function. Various studies have described reduced libido in women during treatment with CPA. The incidence varies between 1 and 25% and seems to be associated with the duration of treatment (Appelt & Strauss, 1984). Loss of libido was reported by 11% of women after the first 3 months of treatment, increasing to 33% after 9 months. This is important because typically therapeutic benefit only starts to be seen with CPA treatment after 3 months. Appelt and Strauss (1984) obtained details of sexual function in hirsute women both before and during CPA therapy. Before treatment, 21% of women were classified by these researchers as having sexual dysfunction (including orgasmic dysfunction, lack of sexual enjoyment and dyspareunia). During treatment this increased to 44% and reached 61% in women in a stable relationship.

It should also be noted that untreated hirsutism *per se* is associated with a reduction in libido. Many hirsute women are also overweight and concerned about their body image compared with an idealised portrait of femininity as depicted in the media (Dixon, Hicks & Chapman, 1991).

CPA was assessed in a group of male paedophiles and was associated with reduced sexual thoughts, decrease in frequency and pleasure of masturbation and diminished sexual frustration. Serum testosterone levels were reduced during drug therapy (Cooper *et al.*, 1992).

Flutamide

Flutamide is a non-steroidal pure antiandrogen that has been used in the treatment of prostatic carcinoma. It acts by inhibiting androgen uptake or inhibiting the binding of androgen to its receptor. One study (Pavone-Macaluso *et al.*, 1990) showed that flutamide did not reduce libido or sexual potency in a group of men with advanced prostatic carcinoma. Another group using flutamide for the same indication showed that it reduced libido in only 20% of the men treated (Johansson *et al.*, 1987). In contrast, a Canadian study (Rousseau *et al.*, 1988) in which complete androgen blockade was obtained by associating flutamide with a GnRH agonist showed that 70% of patients noticed a major reduction in their interest in sexual intercourse during treatment. Only 19% were able to maintain erection during intercourse compared with 56% before treatment. The sexual dysfunction was so marked that the authors suggested that this combination would constitute a useful treatment for sexual offenders.

Finasteride

Finasteride is an inhibitor of 5α-reductase and so it inhibits the conversion of testosterone to dihydrotestosterone, the active form within tissues. It is used in the management of benign prostatic hypertrophy. As an androgen inhibitor it is associated with reduced libido, erectile dysfunction and also produces a reduction in the volume of the seminal ejaculate. The Committee on Safety of Medicines in the UK has reported 800 adverse drug reactions in 65 000 patients who have been prescribed finasteride. The most common adverse reactions (84) were the sexual effects described above (Anon., 1995). Finasteride is excreted in semen and can potentially exert an antiandrogenic effect on the genitalia of male fetuses, so condoms should be used by men whose partners are pregnant or who could become pregnant.

Cimetidine

This is discussed in Chapter 7.

Miscellaneous hormones

Bromocriptine

Bromocriptine is a dopamine agonist widely used in the treatment of hyperprolactinaemia. This disorder is characterised by amenorrhoea and galactorrhoea in women and impotence in males. Infertility is a common presentation of hyperprolactinaemia. Therapy with bromocriptine is generally highly effective in suppressing the elevated prolactin levels and this is associated with a return to normal menstruation in females (secondary to restoration of ovulation) and return to normal sexual function in men (Johnston *et al.*, 1983). Bromocriptine has also been used to restore normal sexual function to uraemic men undergoing haemodialysis, who are frequently affected by reduced libido and potency disorders (Bommer *et al.*, 1979).

In Parkinson's disease, however, the use of bromocriptine has been reported to induce impotence. Cleeves and Findley described four patients who developed erectile dysfunction while being treated with bromocriptine. In one 59-year-old man this was paradoxically associated with increased sexual desire (Cleeves & Findley, 1987). The sexual dysfunction was reversible in all patients either by reducing the dose of bromocriptine or by partial or complete substitution with levodopa. The combination of bromocriptine and levodopa was thought to be responsible for the development of hypersexuality in another case report of drug treatment in Parkinson's disease (Vogel & Schiffter, 1983).

Gonadotrophin-releasing hormone

GnRH is administered to men who have hypogonadism secondary to hypothalamo-pituitary deficiency. It acts by stimulating the pituitary gland to produce gonadotrophins. Two cases of priapism have been reported in 51 hypogonadal men receiving this therapy, presumably as a consequence of rapid increases in testosterone production by the testes (Whalen *et al.*, 1991). Priapism has also been recorded following testosterone therapy (Key *et al.*, 1989; Whalen *et al.*, 1991) and tamoxifen, which by stimulating gonandotrophins would also be expected to increase serum testosterone levels (Fernando & Tobias, 1989).

References

Anon. (1991). Diethylstilboestrol – effects of exposure in utero. *Drug and Therapeutics Bulletin*, 29, 49–50.

Anon. (1995). Finasteride (Proscar). *Current Problems in Pharmacovigilance*, 21, 3.

Appelt, H. & Strauss, B. (1984). Effects of antiandrogen treatment on the sexuality of women with hyperandrogenism. *Psychotherapy and Psychosomatics*, 42, 177–81.

Bibbo, M., Gill, W. B., Azizi, F., Blough, R., Fang, V. S., Rosenfield, R. L, Schumacher, G. F. B., Sleeper, K., Sonek, M. G. & Wied, G. L. (1977). Follow-up study of male and female offspring of DES-exposed mothers. *Obstetrics and Gynaecology*, 49, 1–8.

Bommer, J., Ritz, E., del Pozo, E. & Bommer, G. (1979). Improved sexual function in male haemodialysis patients on bromocriptine. *Lancet*, ii, 496–7.

Buttram, V. C., Reiter, R. C. & Ward, S. (1985). Treatment of endometriosis with danazol: report of a 6 year prospective study. *Fertility and Sterility*, 43, 353–60.

Candiani, G. B., Fedele, L., Vercellini, P., Bianchi, S. & Arcaini, L. (1990). Medical management of mild endometriosis associated with infertility. In *Endometriosis*, ed. R. W. Shaw, pp. 119– 29. Carnforth: Parthenon Publishing.

Cleeves, L. & Findley, L. J. (1987). Bromocriptine-induced impotence in Parkinson's disease. *British Medical Journal*, 295, 367–8.

Cooper, A. J., Sandhu, S., Losztyn, S. & Cernovsky, Z. (1992). A double-blind controlled trial of medroxyprogesterone acetate and cyproterone acetate with seven pedophiles. *Canadian Journal of Psychiatry*, 37, 687–93.

Dixon, J. E., Hicks, B. H. & Chapman, M. G. (1991). Psychological morbidity of hirsute women. *Journal of Obstetrics and Gynaecology*, 11, 198–203.

Emens, J. M. (1994). Continuing problems with diethylstilboestrol. *British Journal of Obstetrics and Gynaecology*, 101, 748–50.

Eri, L. M. & Tveter, K. J. (1994). Safety, side effects and patient acceptance of the luteinising hormone releasing hormone agonist leuprolide in treatment of benign prostatic hyperplasia. *Journal of Urology*, 152, 448–52.

Fernando, I. N. & Tobias, J. S. (1989). Priapism in a patient on tamoxifen. *Lancet*, i, 436.

Friedl, K. E. (1990). Reappraisal of the health risks associated with the use of high doses of oral and injectable androgenic steroids. *Nida Research Monograph*, 102, 142–77.

Gill, W. B, Schumacher, G. F., Bibbo, M., Straus, F.H. & Schoenberg, H.W. (1979). Association of diethylstilboestrol exposure in utero with cryptorchidism, testicular hypoplasia and semen abnormalities, *Journal of Urology*, 122, 36–9.

Graham, C. A. & Sherwin, B. B. (1993). The relationship between mood and sexuality in women using an oral contraceptive as a treatment for premenstrual symptoms. *Psychoneuroendocrinology*, 18, 273–81.

Johansson, J. E., Andersson, S. O., Beckman, K. W., Lingardh, G. & Zador, G. (1987). Clinical evaluation of flutamide and estramustine as initial treatment of metastatic carcinoma of prostate. *Urology*, 29, 55–9.

Johnston, D. G, Prescott, R. W. G., Kendall-Taylor, P., Hall, K., Crombie, A. L., Hall, R., McGregor, A., Watson, M. J. & Cook, D. B. (1983). Hyperprolactinaemia; long term effects of bromocriptine. *American Journal of Medicine*, 75, 868–74.

Kane, F. J. (1976). Evaluation of emotional reactions to oral contraceptive use. *American Journal of Obstetrics and Gynecology*, 126, 968–72.

Key, L. L., Myers, M. C., Kroovand, R. L. & Kelly, W. S. (1989). Priapism following testosterone therapy for delayed puberty. *American Journal of Diseases of Children*, 143, 116–20.

Koutsilieris, M., Faure, N., Tolis, G., Laroche, B., Robert, G. & Ackman, C. F. D. (1986). Objective response and disease outcome in 59 patients with stage D2 prostatic cancer treated with either buserelin or orchidectomy. *Urology*, 27, 221–8.

Marshall, E. (1988). The drug of champions. *Science*, 242, 183–4.

Moss, H. B., Panzak, G. L. & Tarter, R. E. (1993). Sexual functioning of male anabolic steroid abusers. *Archives of Sexual Behaviour*, 22, 1–12.

Palanca, E. & Juco, W. (1977). Conservative treatment of benign prostatic hyperplasia. *Current Medical Research and Opinion*. 4, 513–20.

Pardthaisong, T. (1984). Return of fertility after use of the injectable contraceptive Depoprovera: up-dated data analysis. *Journal of Biosocial Science*, 16, 23–34.

Pavone-Macaluso, M., Serretta, V., Daricello, G., Pavone, C., Cacciatore, M., Romano, C. & Cavallo, N. (1990). Is there a role for pure antiandrogens in the treatment of advanced prostatic cancer. *Progress in Clinical and Biological Research*, 350, 149–57.

Pope, H. G. & Katz, D. L. (1988). Affective and psychotic symptoms associated with anabolic steroid use. *American Journal of Psychiatry*, 145, 487–90.

Rousseau, L., Dupont, A., Labrie, F. & Couture, M. (1988). Sexuality changes in prostate cancer patients receiving antihormonal therapy combining the antiandrogen flutamide with medical (LHRH agonist) or surgical castration. *Archives of Sexual Behaviour*, 17, 87–98.

Senekjian, E. K., Potkul, R. K., Frey, K. & Herbst, A. L. (1988). Infertility among daughters either exposed or not exposed to diethylstilboestrol. *American Journal of Obstetrics and Gynecology*, 158, 493–8.

Shaw, R. W. (1988). LHRH analogues in the treatment of endometriosis–comparative results with other treatments. *Clinical Obstetrics and Gynaecology*, 2, 659–75.

Shaw, R. W. (1992). An open randomised comparative study of the effect of goserelin depot and danazol in the treatment of endometriosis. *Fertility and Sterility*, 58, 265–72.

Stenchever, M. A., Williamson, R. A., Leonard, J., Karp, L. E., Ley, B., Shy, K. & Smith, D. (1981). Possible relationship between in utero diethylstilboestrol exposure and male infertility. *American Journal of Obstetrics and Gynecology*, 140, 186–91.

Thibaut, F., Cordier, B., Kuhn, J. M. (1993). Effect of a long-lasting gonadotrophin hormone releasing-hormone agonist in six cases of severe male paraphilia. *Acta Psychiatrica Scandinavica*, 87, 445–50.

Uzych, L. (1992). Anabolic-androgenic steroids and psychiatric-related effects: a review. *Canadian Journal of Psychiatry*, 37, 23–8.

Van der Zon, P. (1990). Safety of testosterone enanthate. *Lancet*, 336, 1517–18.

Vogel, H. P. & Schiffter, R. (1983). Hypersexuality–a complication of dopaminergic therapy in Parkinson's disease. *Pharmacopsychiatria*, 16, 107–10.

Whalen, R. K., Whitcomb, R. W., Crowley, W. F. Jr & McGovern, F. J. (1991). Priapism in hypogonadal men receiving gonadotropin releasing hormone. *Journal of Urology*, 145, 1051–2.

World Health Organisation Task Force on Methods for Regulation of Male Fertility (1990). Contraceptive efficacy of testosterone-induced azoospermia in normal men. *Lancet*, 336, 955–9.

6
Antibiotics

Sulphonamides

Sulphasalazine

Sulphasalazine has been used in the treatment of inflammatory bowel disease since 1942, although the first reports of sperm toxicity only appeared in 1979. Sulphasalazine is taken orally and reaches the colon intact. As a result of the action of colonic bacteria, the compound is split into its constituents sulphapyridine and 5-aminosalicylic acid. It is useful to follow the sulphasalazine story in some detail. It is one of the few drugs for which clinical observation of reproductive side effects has led to detailed study of the underlying mechanisms responsible for the side effects. This has resulted in identification of the toxic component and a change in the pharmacological formulation.

Two separate reports in 1979 drew attention to men with inflammatory bowel disease presenting with infertility while being treated with long-term sulphasalazine. Levi *et al.* (1979) noted reduced sperm count and motility that improved after withdrawal of the drug. Three of the four men fathered children when sulphasalazine was discontinued. The sperm abnormalities returned when the drug was reintroduced. Toth described 10 subfertile men on sulphasalazine. Six stopped treatment and their wives all conceived. He also noted a particular sperm morphological abnormality consisting of a ballooned enlarged sperm with a pale staining head. This appearance was thought to result from immaturity of the sperm coupled with osmotic damage to the membrane structures (Toth, 1979a,b). Others also described large numbers of immature sperm, suggesting a toxic action on sperm maturation. At this time, it was also postulated that the adverse effect could be related to the antiprostaglandin action of sulphasalazine, as prostaglandins are thought to be implicated in sperm motility (Traub, Thompson & Carville, 1979).

The above reports were in men presenting to fertility clinics. Later, abnormal semen analyses were also found in 18 of 21 men attending gastrointestinal outpatient clinics (Birnie, McLeod, & Watkinson, 1981).

As a consequence, the temporal relationship between sulphasalazine administration and fertility was investigated. The sperm of men currently receiving sulphasalazine was compared with that of men who had recently discontinued therapy and men who had stopped therapy more than 2 months previously. All men on sulphasalazine had severe reductions in sperm count and motility as well as an increase in the number of abnormal sperm forms, as might be expected. However within 2 months there was recovery of count and motility to normal values, although the morphological abnormalities persisted. Gonadotrophin and testosterone levels within the blood were within the normal range, confirming a direct toxic effect on spermatogenesis (Toovey *et al.*, 1981). Other studies have confirmed the existence of large headed sperm and their persistence after other parameters of semen analysis have returned to normal following discontinuation of sulphasalazine (Riley *et al.*, 1987).

In 1984, an important paper was published confirming the rapid reversibility of sulphasalazine-induced sperm damage (O'Morain *et al.*, 1984). The median time to conception in couples after the man had discontinued treatment was 2.5 months. Men who were genetically slow acetylators had significantly lower sperm counts than fast acetylators. Sulphapyridine is metabolised by acetylation so that slow acetylators will have higher blood levels of this metabolite than the fast acetylators. An interesting aspect of this work was the parallel studies performed in rats.

Sulphasalazine was found to induce reversible male infertility in rats that was dose related (this helps to explain the more pronounced effects of sulphasalazine in human males who were slow acetylators). Examination of the rat testicles showed no changes in treated animals, providing further evidence that the adverse effect is on sperm maturation. Perhaps the most important finding was the results of the studies when rats were treated with sulphasalazine, its metabolite sulphapyridine or the therapeutically active form 5-aminosalicylic acid. Both sulphasalazine and sulphapyridine produced infertility, but 5-aminosalicylic acid had no spermatoxic effect. Similar results were seen in infertile men when their therapy was switched from sulphasalazine to 5-aminosalicylic acid (Cann & Holdsworth, 1984). This finding ruled out the possibility of sperm toxicity occurring as a result of the antiprostaglandin action of sulphasalazine, as this activity is induced by 5-aminosalicylic acid.

Sulphasalazine may not be the only factor reducing fertility in men with inflammatory bowel disease. There is some tentative evidence that Crohn's disease may impair the fertility of men independent of sulphasalazine use (Burnell *et al.*, 1986). This could be related to decreased nutritional status (Farthing & Dawson, 1983), although this is disputed.

More recent studies have attempted to assess more subtle defects induced by sulphasalazine on sperm function. Notably one report described a patient taking sulphasalazine who had normal conventional semen parameters but abnormal results in the hamster egg penetration test. When the therapy was changed to 5-aminosalicylic acid, the hamster egg penetration test result became normal. Another group looked at the production of reactive oxygen species (superoxide radicals) by the sperm of men with inflammatory bowel disease taking sulphasalazine and again after changing to 5-aminosalicylic acid (Wu, Aitken & Ferguson, 1989). The production of excessive levels of reactive oxygen species may be responsible for defective sperm function in previously unexplained cases of infertility. However, levels of reactive oxygen species in men on salazopyrin were in the normal range.

Co-trimoxazole

Co-trimoxazole is a fixed ratio mixture of trimethoprim and the sulphonamide sulphamethoxazole. A report from India published in 1978 noted that 14 men from a group of 40 treated with co-trimoxazole for suspected genitourinary infection showed a reduction of sperm count within a month of starting treatment. The authors proposed that the trimethoprim moiety may be responsible as it inhibits dihydrofolate reductase which could deprive the rapidly dividing sperm cells of folic acid (Murdia *et al.*, 1978). It was quickly pointed out that although the sperm count dropped in a third of the men it actually rose in another 42% and was stable in the remainder. Furthermore, the sperm decreases were all evident 1 month after initiation of treatment, which is too short for an effect on spermatogenesis. This evidence per se is not sufficient to implicate co-trimoxazole as a toxic agent for sperm.

Nitrofurans

Niridazole

Niridazole is a nitrothiazole derivative related to metronidazole and is widely used in some countries for the treatment of schistosomiasis. In rodent species, it has been found to affect spermatogenesis during meiosis. A study of 25 men with bilharzia in Egypt showed that a 10 day course of treatment depressed semen volume and sperm count and motility 1 week after cessation of treatment. This persisted 3 months after treatment was discontinued. Testicular biopsy at 1 week in eight men showed focal germinal cell hypoplasia and/or spermatocyte arrest. At 3 months, repeat testicular biopsy in these men showed normal spermatogenesis in six but persistant abnormalities in the remaining two subjects. (El-Beheiry, Kamel & Gad, 1982).

Nitrofurantoin

Early studies in rats showed that nitrofurans including nitrofurantoin produced transient spermatogenic arrest at the stage of the primary spermatocyte. In a clinical study performed in 1956 (and unlikely to be repeated) prisoners and medical student 'volunteers' were given a 14 day course of nitrofurantoin at a daily dose of 10 mg/kg. Semen samples were obtained pre- and post-treatment. Testicular biopsies were performed pre- and post-treatment in one third of medical students and all prisoners! The results were difficult to interpret. The majority of volunteers showed no changes in sperm count or testicular histology. In approximately 30% of the subjects a temporary decrease was recorded in sperm count but without accompanying histological abnormalities (Nelson & Bunge, 1957).

The recommended daily dose of nitrofurantoin is now approximately 5 mg/kg and this compound is sometimes used for long-term antibiotic therapy. No clinical studies have reported an adverse fertility effect at this dose, but Schlegel and co-workers recommend avoidance of nitrofurantoin as long-term suppressive therapy in men 'interested in fertility' (Schlegel, Chang & Marshall, 1991). Certainly if a man has a suboptimal semen analysis on nitrofurantoin, withdrawal of therapy would be a sensible first-line measure.

Ketoconazole

The data sheet for the antifungal drug ketoconazole notes that gynaecomastia and oligospermia have been reported in rare instances. A possible explanation for this can be provided from a study performed in five healthy volunteers who each received a single oral dose of 400 mg of ketoconazole. The levels of total and free testosterone fell sharply, reaching a nadir of approximately 30% below baseline levels within 4 to 6 hours of drug ingestion. The decrease was thought to be caused by reduced testosterone synthesis as it is known that spermatogenesis is regulated by intratesticular levels of testosterone. The authors state that this mechanism could be responsible for the loss of libido and potency seen in men on ketoconazole, although no data are provided on the incidence of these sexual dysfunctions (Schürmeyer & Niesschlag, 1982). Furthermore, the drug manufacturers acknowledge the transient fall in testosterone levels in the data sheet but note that during long-term therapy testosterone levels are not usually significantly different from controls.

Tetracyclines

Tetracyclines do not appear to affect spermatogenesis, but some forms may have a direct toxic effect on mature sperm. *Chlortetracycline* has deleterious effects on human sperm at concentrations of 100 mg/l and minocycline has been found to be toxic to bull sperm. Tetracycline hydrochloride is not toxic to ejaculated human sperm at concentrations of $4 \mu g/10^6$ sperm, but it has not been tested at higher concentrations. Schlegel *et al.*, (1991) suggest that when these drugs are used to treat genito urinary infections any adverse effect may be outweighed by the beneficial effect of eradicating infection and inflammatory cells from the ejaculate. In men requiring long-term antibiotic administration, the type of antibiotic should be judiciously chosen. However, it must be noted that the few studies published that do demonstrate sperm toxicity with tetracyclines were performed between 1955 and 1975 and no recent evidence substantiates toxic effects in humans at therapeutic doses.

Demeclocycline

A single case report describes a 22-year-old man who, after several years of treatment with tetracycline for acne, changed to demeclocycline. He complained of decreased libido at doses between 300 to 600 mg/day. The symptoms resolved within a week of discontinuing the drug (Biro & Price, 1974).

Macrolides

The macrolides, which include *erythromycin* and *spiramycin*, have no effect on human or animal sperm at long-term exposure to therapeutic drug concentrations. However short-term exposure at high doses may impair sperm motility. Erythromycin administered at therapeutic levels decreased the frequency of mitotic division in rat testes. Based on this data, Schlegel *et al.* (1991) suggest that macrolides might impair fertility in men during the period of drug administration.

Aminoglycosides

Gentamicin appears to have negative effects on spermatogenesis in humans and animals. Men receiving gentamicin before prostatic surgery developed meoitic arrest at the primary spermatocyte stage. Unfortunately no information is provided on the incidence of this effect nor the reason why the men were having prostate surgery (Timmermans, 1974). Similar findings were reported in rats treated for 8 days with therapeutic doses of gentamicin. In one study reported in the 1970s, *neomycin* used in the treatment of men with chronic inflammatory conditions of the genitourinary tract had an adverse effect on sperm count and motility. Confirmatory results were provided by the use of therapeutic doses of neomycin in rats, which developed spermatogenic arrest after 20 days of treatment (Schlegel *et al.*, 1991).

Antivirals

Amantadine

Amantadine is an antiviral agent also occasionally used in the treatment of Parkinson's disease. Circumstantial evidence for an antifertility effect is provided in a case report from an *in vitro* fertilisation (IVF) unit. This involved a couple who had undergone four cycles of *in vitro* fertilisation. Oocyte fertilisation occurred in three of the four cycles with at least 50% of the oocytes fertilising. In the remaining cycle there was no fertilisation of any of six eggs despite apparently healthy looking oocytes. In this cycle, the husband had taken amantadine for antiviral prophylaxis for 2 weeks before the fertilisation cycle. All sperm parameters appeared normal but electron microscopic examination of the oocyte 24 hours after exposure to sperm showed that sperm although able to attach to the zona pellucida (the outer coat surrounding the oocyte) were not able to penetrate through it (Cowan *et al.*, 1988). It must be noted, however, that there are several reasons for experiencing complete failure of fertilisation in an *in vitro* fertilisation programme.

References

Birnie, G. G., McLeod, T. I. F. & Watkinson, G. (1981). Incidence of sulphasalazine induced male infertility. *Gut*, 22, 452–5.

Biro, L. & Price, E. (1974). Demeclocycline hydrochloride and diminished sex drive. *Archives of Dermatology*, 110, 637.

Burnell, D., Mayberry, J., Calcraft, B. J., Morris, J. S. & Rhodes, J. (1986). Male infertility in Crohns disease. *Postgraduate Medical Journal*, 62, 269–72.

Cann, P. A. & Holdsworth, C. D. (1984). Reversal of male infertility on changing treatment from sulphasalazine to 5-aminosalicylic acid. *Lancet*, i, 1119.

Cowan, B. D., Lucas, J. A. III, Sopelak, V. M. & Lockard, V. (1988). *Journal of In Vitro Fertilisation and Embryo Transfer*, 5, 282–5.

El-Beheiry, A. H., Kamel, M. N. & Gad, A. (1982). Niridazole and fertility in bilharzial men. *Archives of Andrology*, 8, 297–300.

Farthing, M. J. G. & Dawson, A. M., (1983). Impaired semen quality in Crohns disease–drugs, ill health or undernutrition. *Scandinavian Journal of Gastroenterology*, 18, 57–60.

Levi, A. J., Fisher, A. M., Hughes, L. & Hendry, W. F. (1979). Male infertility due to sulphasalazine. *Lancet*, ii, 276–8.

Murdia, A., Mathur, V., Kothari, L. K. & Singh, K. P. (1978). Sulpha–trimethoprim combinations and male fertility. *Lancet* , ii, 375–6.

Nelson, W. O. & Bunge, R. G. (1957). The effect of therapeutic dosages of nitrofurantoin (furadantin) upon spermatogenesis in man. *Journal of Urology*, 77, 275–81.

O'Morain, C., Smethurst, P., Doré, C. J. & Levi, A. J. (1984). Reversible male infertility due to sulphasalazine: studies in men and rats. *Gut*, 25, 1078–84.

Riley, S. A., Lecarpentier, J., Mani, V., Goodman, M. J., Mandal, B. K. & Turnberg, L. A. (1987). Sulphasalazine induced seminal abnormalities in ulcerative colitis: results of mesalazine substitution. *Gut*, 28, 1008–12.

Schlegel, P. N., Chang, T. S. K. & Marshall, F. F. (1991). Antibiotics: potential hazards to male infertility. *Fertility and Sterility*, 55, 235–42.

Schürmeyer, T. & Niesschlag, E. (1982). Ketoconazole-induced drop in serum and saliva testosterone. *Lancet*, ii, 1098.

Timmermans, L. (1974). Influence of antibiotics on spermatogenesis. *Journal of Urology*, 112, 348–9.

Toovey, S., Hudson, E., Hendry, W. F. & Levi, A. J. (1981). Sulphasalazine and male infertility: reversibility and possible mechanism. *Gut*, 22, 445–51.

Toth, A. (1979a). Male infertility due to sulphasalazine. *Lancet*, ii, 904.

Toth, A. (1979b). Reversible toxic effect of salicyclazosulfapyridine on semen quality. *Fertility and Sterility*, 31, 538–40.

Traub, A. I., Thompson, W. & Carville, J. (1979). Male infertility due to sulphasalazine. *Lancet*, ii, 639–40.

Wu, F. C. W., Aitken, R. J. & Ferguson, A. (1989). Inflammatory bowel disease and male infertility: effects of sulfasalazine and 5-aminosalicylic acid on sperm fertilising capacity and reactive oxygen species generation. *Fertility and Sterility*, 52, 842–5.

7
Miscellaneous drugs

Gastrointestinal drugs

Cimetidine

Cimetidine was first introduced in the USA for the treatment of duodenal ulcer in 1978. It is a histamine (H_2) receptor antagonist that was generally thought to be well tolerated apart from the known occurrence of gynaecomastia. In 1979, however, several case reports appeared in the UK and the USA suggesting that cimetidine was associated with impotence (Wolfe, 1979; Peden *et al.*, 1979). It was suggested that because minor elevations of gonadotrophins, testosterone and prolactin were found this side effect may have an endocrine basis. However, these hormonal disturbances were mild and unlikely to influence sexual function directly. A study in the USA of seven men taking cimetidine reported an average reduction in sperm count of 43% after 6 weeks of therapy, although sperm concentrations remained within the normal range (Van Thiel *et al.*, 1979). Furthermore, although there was no difference in basal FSH or LH before or after cimetidine, testosterone levels were higher after treatment. The authors postulated that as cimetidine is an antiandrogen it might be having an atrophic effect on androgen-dependent tissues (similar findings had been recorded in rats given cimetidine).

This study was subsequently criticised on methodological grounds, specifically that spermatogenesis is known to take over 10 weeks whereas the authors were reporting decreased sperm counts after 6 weeks. (White, Gore & Jewell, 1979). A case report has also described rapid and reversible loss of libido in a woman within 3 days of commencing cimetidine (Pierce, 1983). The authors suggested that, as androgens are thought to stimulate libido in women, the antiandrogenic action of cimetidine might have the opposing effect.

Several theoretical mechanisms have been proposed to explain the sexual dysfunction provoked by cimetidine. These include endocrine mechanisms and notably, hyperprolactinaemia. Histamine-mediated release of prolactin is known to occur, so potentially cimetidine might act at this level. However, ranitidine, another H_2 histamine receptor antagonist does not induce hyperprolactinaemia and so any effect of cimetidine on prolactin may not occur via the H_2 histamine receptor (Lardinois & Mazzaferri, 1985). It is also suggested that histamine involvement may operate at a different level. Specifically, histamine has been postulated to act as an inhibitory neurotransmitter that relaxes the smooth muscle of the corpora cavernosa in the penis. This allows blood to enter the penile muscles leading to erection. Chemicals related to cimetidine are known to abolish the relaxant effect of histamine. It is hypothesised that by blocking H_2 histamine receptors on the body of the penis, cimetidine may prevent erection (Adaikan & Karim, 1979). Against this theory, the authors acknowledge that there is no specific evidence to prove that histamine is indeed a neurotransmitter acting on the corpora cavernosa. Furthermore, this theory does not take account of the lack of an adverse effect with ranitidine.

Ranitidine

Ranitidine treatment is not thought to be associated with sexual dysfunction. In view of the known antiandrogenic effects of cimetidine, these have been specifically sought with ranitidine both *in vitro* and *in vivo*. It does not interact with androgen receptors *in vitro* nor produce antiandrogenic effects in laboratory animals. In humans, ranitidine is not associated with changes in testosterone, oestrogens, FSH or LH (Peden & Wormsley, 1983). Most importantly, ranitidine can reverse the antiandrogenic effects produced by cimetidine. The clinical relevance of this is shown in a case report in which a 50 year-old-man taking cimetidine at a dose of 1 g/day for 18 months had developed impotence. His potency recovered completely when therapy was changed to ranitidine; indeed he subsequently developed a sexually transmitted disease (Peden & Wormsley, 1982)!

Long-term effects of ranitidine were studied in 20 men treated for duodenal ulcer with ranitidine or placebo for 12 months. No differences in serum reproductive hormones were recorded between the active treatment group and controls. Sperm count, motility and morphology were similar in both groups. Two patients taking ranitidine had hamster egg penetration tests both before and after therapy and normal results were obtained (Wang *et al.*, 1983).

In view of the apparent lack of sexual side effects of ranitidine compared with cimetidine, consideration should be given to the use of ranitidine in men, all other factors being equal. Certainly, patients on cimetidine should be specifically questioned for adverse sexual side effects.

Metoclopramide

The antiemetic metoclopramide increases gastric motility. It acts centrally to block dopamine receptors and consequently induces hyperprolactinaemia. Prolactin levels rise immediately following the administration of clinical dosages of metoclopramide and sexual side effects related to hyperprolactinaemia have been reported.

At a total dose of 30 mg/day, serum prolactin levels increased tenfold after 1 week in a group of five healthy volunteers. Four men had a reduction in libido and three lost spontaneous erections. All men had decreased volume of seminal fluid and a reduced sperm count after 1 month. Within a week of stopping metoclopramide, prolactin levels had nearly normalised (Falaschi et al., 1978). Case reports have described impotence in patients being treated for nausea and oesophagitis at a dose of 40 mg/day. This was reversible after discontinuation of therapy (Berlin, 1986).

In women, metoclopramide use is associated with galactorrhoea, and amenorrhoea has been reported starting 2 months after initiation of therapy. All these effects are reversible once treatment is stopped (Andersen, Hansen & Madsen, 1981).

Omeprazole

Omeprazole is used in the treatment of reflux oesophagitis and gastric and duodenal ulceration. It inhibits gastric acid production by blocking the hydrogen-potassium adenosine triphosphate enzyme system (the proton pump) of gastric parietal cells. It is not an antiandrogen.

Recently, several reports have described the occurrence of sexual disorders in patients taking omeprazole. The most significant report originates from the WHO Collaborating Centre for International Drug Monitoring and is a collation of cases from several countries (Lindquist & Edwards, 1992). Fifteen men developed impotence after a mean of 4 days treatment with omeprazole at a daily dose of 20–40 mg. Gynaecomastia occurred in 13 men and breast enlargement in two women at these doses. One third of the patients were known to be concomitantly receiving other drugs, although the authors thought that in at least 14 cases there was adequate information to implicate omeprazole directly. It is difficult to postulate a mechanism for the gynaecomastia and impotence, although it has been suggested that inhibition of cytochrome P-450 may be a factor.

In contrast, painful erections have been described in a case report of a 77-year-old man being treated with omeprazole. Erections developed after each tablet and persisted for 36 hours. The patient also took glyceryl trinitrate for angina and had done so for years. Although glyceryl trinitrate is a powerful vasodilator, the authors did not believe it to be the cause of the erections as these did not occur when the omeprazole was withdrawn (Dutertre *et al.*, 1991).

Cardiovascular drugs

Antiarrhythmics

Disopyramide

Disopyramide is used for the prevention and control of a wide variety of cardiac arrhythmias. At least two case reports have described the development of impotence but with no loss of sexual desire in patients on disopyramide. One patient developed impotence on a dose of 300–400 mg disopyramide. At this time plasma disopyramide concentration was 14 µg/ml. The dosage was reduced and full recovery of sexual function occurred when the plasma concentration fell to 3 µg/ml (McHaffie, Guz & Johnston, 1977). In another case, impotence developed in a 35-year-old man within 3 weeks of commencing disopyramide. Six days after withdrawal of the drug, sexual potency returned. Disopyramide was later recommenced because of a recurrence of his ectopic beats and the sexual dysfunction returned (Ahmad, 1980). Both authors suggest that the mechanism of impotence is via the anticholinergic action of disopyramide causing interference with parasympathetic sacral outflow.

Verapamil

Verapamil is a calcium-channel blocker used in the treatment of arrhythmia, angina and mild to moderate hypertension. Its sexual and reproductive effects are described in Chapter 2.

Amiodarone

Amiodarone prolongs the action potential duration in both atrial and ventricular myocardium. Few data are available on this drug. In a study of plasma and red blood cell amiodarone concentrations in 28 patients, it is incidentally mentioned that nine of the patients experienced one or more adverse side effects including anorexia, nausea, marked muscle weakness, unsteady gait and impotence. No further details are given (Heger *et al.*, 1984). In the drug data sheet epididymo-orchitis is mentioned as an occasionally reported unwanted effect. The reasons for this effect are unclear.

Digoxin

Digoxin is a cardiac glycoside that both increases the force of myocardial contractility and reduces myocardial conductivity. Oestrogen-like side effects can occur. The data sheet describes gynaecomastia after long-term administration. In a study of cardiac patients, plasma oestradiol levels were higher and testosterone and LH levels lower in those patients taking digoxin for more than 2 years compared with non-treated control patients. Furthermore, the treated men had a higher incidence of erectile difficulties and a lower frequency of sexual intercourse than untreated controls. The severity of cardiac disease (which in itself can alter sexual function) was comparable in the two groups (Neri *et al.*, 1987). The authors suggest that digoxin or one of its metabolites may have an oestrogenic action on target tissues. Alternatively, it may stimulate the pituitary-adrenal axis to produce more oestrogen. These data are compatible with the hypothesis that the raised oestrogen suppresses pituitary LH by negative feedback and this could lead to hypogonadism and sexual dysfunction.

Hypolipaemics

Clofibrate

Clofibrate, a fibric acid derivative, was one of the earliest effective lipid-lowering agents. Three cases of impotence developing on clofibrate treatment were reported in a group of approximately 100 hyperlipoproteinaemic men during treatment. In two patients, the impotence resolved after withdrawal of treatment. The third patient elected to continue clofibrate treatment. The mechanism of action was unclear although possibly it interferes with androgen metabolism (Schneider & Kaffarnik, 1975). Impotence has also been noted with *bezafibrate*, although in one report a patient who developed impotence on gemfibrozil had no sexual problems on bezafibrate (Bain, Lemon & Jones, 1990).

Gemfibrozil

Gemfibrozil is another fibric acid derivative used in the management of hyperlipidaemia. It is licensed in the UK for the primary prevention of coronary heart disease in men between 40 and 55 years with resistant hyperlipidaemias. Several case reports described the development of impotence within 2 to 4 weeks of commencing gemfibrozil treatment. In addition, at least six other instances had been reported to the CSM by 1992 (Bharani, 1992) The Spanish National Drug Surveillance system was aware of four cases in 1993. One of these patients had also reported impotence on clofibrate (Figueras *et al.*, 1993). Although the incidence of impotence is probably not high, the drug is used in relatively younger, sexually active patients, and it is, therefore, a potentially important side effect. Impotence appears to be reversible once drug therapy is discontinued.

Lovastatin

A case report in 1990 described a 38-year-old man with hypercholesterolaemia treated with lovastatin. He had apparently previously fathered a child. As he was experiencing difficulty fathering another child, a sperm count was performed. The value was very low at 3.2 million/ml. After lovastatin was stopped, the count exceeded 70 million/ml (Hilderbrand & Hepperlen, 1990). The authors described this as a potential adverse effect of lovastatin, but such variability in the sperm count could also be associated with non-drug-related factors.

Vitamins

Etretinate

Etretinate is a vitamin A derivative indicated for the treatment of psoriasis. Isolated reports of erectile dysfunction related to etretinate have been published (Reynolds, 1991). A study investigating sperm during acitretin (a metabolite of etretinate) therapy in both psoriasis patients and healthy volunteers showed no positive or negative influence of treatment for 3 months on any of the sperm parameters measured. Gonadotrophin and testosterone levels in blood were unaffected by therapy (Parsch *et al.*, 1989).

One report described menstrual abnormalities developing in a 34-year-old women on etretinate (Halkier-Sørensen, 1987). Her periods gradually decreased from 5 days of menstrual loss to spotting lasting for only 1 day. This was accompanied by total loss of libido. All symptoms resolved within a few months of finishing treatment. Prior to this episode, the patient had never had menstrual problems. The author of this report comments that several cases of absent or decreased menstrual flow have been described in chronic vitamin A intoxication. The mechanism is uncertain.

Isotretinoin

A recent case report describes the development of ejaculatory failure in a 29-year-old man on 1 mg/kg per day of isotretinoin (Coleman & MacDonald, 1994). Sexual intercourse occurred daily both before and during therapy, but within 1 week of commencing treatment he could only ejaculate occasionally although there was no problem with erection. Two other cases of ejaculatory failure had been reported to the drug manufacturers. The authors postulated that as isotretinoin is associated with a general reduction in body secretions it may be having a similar effect on the goblet cells of the prostate and seminal vesicles, which are responsible for producing 80% of seminal fluid volume. The manufacturers had also received 150 notifications of problems with the reproductive tract in men taking isotretinoin including 'potency disorders, reduced fertility and local inflammation/discomfort'. Some of these, of course, may have been unrelated to the drug administration.

Vitamin B_6

Pyridoxine, vitamin B_6, is an essential vitamin that acts as a coenzyme in many decarboxylation and transamination reactions. It is sometimes used in the management of premenstrual syndrome but other uses have included treatment of carpal tunnel syndrome and homocystinuria. Typical doses in humans would be 100 mg/day although higher doses are sometimes used. In a study in rats, it was found that daily administration of megadoses of pyridoxine of greater than 500 mg/kg per day induced severe testicular atrophy and marked reductions in sperm count (Mori *et al.*, 1989). However, this dose would equate with a human dose of 1500 to 2000 mg/day. There have been no reports of defective spermatogenesis in humans taking pyridoxine.

Vitamin C

A letter published in the Lancet in 1973 raised the hypothesis that self administration of high doses of vitamin C as prophylaxis against the common cold could be a cause of infertility in women (Briggs, 1973a). The author offered no data but suggested that vitamin C could act locally within cervical mucus to disorganise the orderly arrangement of molecules. It is known that the linear arrangement of these molecules into channels promotes the passage of sperm. Subsequent to this hypothesis, several letters were published in the Lancet which both supported and opposed the hypothesis. One letter reported four women taking vitamin C at doses of 2 to 4 g per day. All had previously had children but failed to conceive whilst on therapy for between 6 and 17 months. Two then conceived within 3 months of stopping the vitamins (Briggs, 1973b). However, another publication described a personal series of 3000 patients amassed over 20 years who had received large doses of vitamin C with no apparent reduction in fertility (Hoffer, 1973). No evidence has subsequently emerged to support the concept that vitamin C causes infertility.

Analgesics

Non-steroidal anti-inflammatory drugs

Naproxen and indomethacin

Ejaculatory dysfunction was reported in a 66-year-old man treated with naproxen at a dose of 250 mg three times a day for arthralgia. He was also taking aspirin and hydrochlorthiazide. The symptoms started 1 week after he commenced naproxen and resolved 1 week after stopping it. While continuing the other drugs, he agreed to a rechallenge test. The day after naproxen was readministered he was again unable to ejaculate (Wei & Hood, 1980). It was speculated that the ejaculatory function was related to prostaglandin inhibition.

Decreased libido and impotence were reported in a 60-year-old man 2 to 3 weeks following the initiation of therapy with 75 mg of a sustained release indomethacin preparation. The patient discontinued therapy himself and reported that symptoms resolved within 1 week. Interestingly, this patient was then treated with naproxen and had no further sexual dysfunction, although he took naproxen only intermittently. The authors also presumed that the impotence was caused by prostaglandin inhibition as prostaglandins have been shown to be directly involved in the control of human penile tumescence and erection (Miller, Rogers & Swee, 1989).

In females, it has been shown that prostaglandin synthetase inhibitors taken at midcycle can inhibit ovulation (Killick & Elstein, 1987). Volunteer women received either indomethacin, *azapropazone* or placebo control. Follicular rupture was monitored by serial ultrasound. Lack of follicular rupture occurred in 10% of the control cycles, 50% of azapropazone-treated cycles and 100% of indomethacin-treated cycles. The lack of ovulation was so consistent with indomethacin that the authors suggested that it could be considered as a method of contraception, although probably the side effect profile made this impracticable. They also suggested the probability of a dose-dependent response, as azapropazone is a weaker prostaglandin inhibitor than indomethacin. This effect is almost certainly the result of prostaglandin deficiency, as prostaglandin $F_{2\alpha}$ mediates rupture of the ovarian follicle in response to the LH surge at midcycle.

We have previously reported a possible effect of this in clinical practice. A 31-year-old woman with rheumatoid arthritis, being treated with penicillamine and naproxen at a dose of 1g/day, presented with infertility. She appeared to be ovulating, based on measurements of progesterone levels in the second half of her menstrual cycle. However serial ultrasound scanning of her ovary in three successive cycles showed that, despite normal development of the ovarian follicle, follicular rupture was not occurring. Naproxen was withdrawn and prednisolone administered with the penicillamine. Six months later ovulation was seen to have occurred at the time of a laparoscopy and she conceived shortly afterwards (Kennedy, Forman & Barlow, 1991).

In view of these findings, the stronger non-steroidal anti-inflammatory drugs should probably be avoided in women trying to conceive and certainly during the few days around ovulation.

Other drugs

Nasal vasoconstrictors

Pseudoephedrine, phenylpropanolamine, phenylephrine and *oxymetazoline* are nasal decongestants used for 'chronic sinusitis'. They act by causing arterial constriction. One group reported 16 men aged between 30 and 66 years who developed impotence following chronic ingestion of these drugs for between 1 and 40 years (Zorgniotti, Rossman & Claire, 1987). Some did have other risk factors for impotence, including hypertension, smoking, etc. The authors proposed that as erection requires arterial vasodilatation, chronic arterial vasoconstriction would predispose patients to erectile impotence, particularly as there were many similarities between the corpora cavernosum and the nasal turbinate. Further support for this hypothesis is provided by the converse situation as, in some men, significant nasal congestion occurs during sexual excitement.

Aminocaproic acid

Aminocaproic acid is a fibrinolytic inhibitor that has been used in haemophiliacs to decrease bleeding following tooth extractions. Four of

25 patients enrolled in a study for this indication spontaneously reported absent ejaculation without loss of erection. A fifth patient receiving aminocaproic acid but who was not in the study had a similar complaint. The problem arose 24 hours following drug administration and the earliest resumption of normal ejaculation occurred 6 hours after the last dose was administered. No mechanism was proposed to explain the phenomenon but the authors pointed out that 'dry ejaculation' with other drugs was often secondary to retrograde ejaculation (Evans & Aledort, 1978).

Colchicine

Colchicine was originally used as a treatment for gout but since the mid-1970s it has been used for the long-term prevention of attacks of familial mediterranean fever (FMF). This disease affects both sexes in the Middle East and North Africa and is characterised by attacks of fever, peritonitis, pleuritis and arthritis. Continuous prophylaxis with colchicine is effective. FMF itself is associated with infertility in women because of pelvic adhesions and ovulatory disturbances. It does not seem to be a cause of fertility problems in males.

Colchicine interacts with microtubules within cells and inhibits mitosis. Large doses given to experimental male animals destroys the germinal epithelium in the testes and leads to azoospermia. The doses used in the animal systems were 30 to 50 times higher than the equivalent therapeutic dose in humans. An isolated report has described reversible azoospermia in a man treated with colchicine at a dose of 1.2 mg/per day for 3 years (Merlin, 1972). However, a systematic study of colchicine given to seven normal volunteers showed no influence on sperm or hormonal values (Bremner & Paulsen, 1976). Two more recent reviews have retrospectively analysed fertility in male and female patients with FMF both during and without treatment (Ehrenfeld *et al.*, 1986, 1987). Four of 19 males had fertility problems while on colchicine therapy although three of them were able to father children whilst off therapy. Three of the four men with fertility problems had normal sperm counts and motility, but the results of hamster egg penetration tests suggested defective sperm function. The fourth patient already had two children, but a sperm test while he was taking colchicine revealed azoospermia. The authors took this as evidence that up to 20% of patients on long-term colchicine may develop fertility problems. There was no convincing evidence that colchicine caused infertility in a group of 36 women being treated for FMF.

Carbonic anhydrase inhibitors

Carbonic anhydrase inhibitors (CAI) are used for the management of glaucoma, although some are also indicated for the management of water retention and familial cerebellar ataxia. The main reporting of side effects is from ophthalmological practice. The National Registry of Drug Induced Ocular Side Effects in the USA reported 39 cases of decreased libido in patients on CAI. The preparations used included *acetazolamide, dichlorphenamide* and *methazolamide*. In 24 of the cases, the patients had actually demanded of their doctors whether the drug was having an effect on their sexual function. Most patients were taking other drugs concomitantly. In all cases, the symptoms resolved on stopping the CAI. Twelve patients restarted the drug and this was followed by another reduction in libido. Three patients also developed impotence which was reversible. The authors thought that the loss of libido was part of the general malaise and depression that are well recognised side effects of CAI, rather than being a direct drug effect (Wallace *et al.*, 1979).

A later paper described four men treated with either acetazolamide or methazolamide. Between 4 days and 4 weeks later all patients had developed impotence that was not accompanied by loss of libido. All patients were also taking other drugs, in particular timolol, which is also known to be associated with impotence. However, in three patients the impotence resolved within 2 days to 1 week of stopping CAI, despite continuation of timolol. In the remaining case, the impotence resolved on reducing the dose of acetazolamide from 1000 mg/day to 500 mg/day. In this report, as the impotence was not related to lack of libido it was thought unlikely that it was secondary to a general depression (Epstein, Allen & Lunde, 1987). The possibility of adrenal hyperfunction being implicated was discussed as CAI are known to produce this state and a previous case report had described the occurrence of hirsutism in a 2-year-old patient after treatment with acetazolamide.

Interferon

Interferon α-2a was used in the treatment of a 37-year-old man with chronic myelogenous leukaemia. He did not experience any sexual side effects until the dose reached 9 million IU/day. He then developed erectile impotence, which did not resolve until the drug was stopped. He was not taking any other medication. It was proposed that interferon α-2a could produce impotence either by inhibition of the parasympathetic nervous system or by enhancement of prolactin secretion, although no evidence was presented to support these hypotheses (Alvarez, Sacristan & Alsar, 1991).

References

Adaikan, P. G., Karim, S. M. M. (1979). Male sexual function during treatment with cimetidine. *British Medical Journal*, 1, 1282–3.

Ahmad, S. (1980). Disopyramide and impotence, *Southern Medical Journal*, 73, 958.

Alvarez, J. S., Sacristan, J. A., Alsar, M. J. (1991) Interferon α-2a-induced impotence. *DICP, Annals of Pharmacotherapy*, 25, 1397.

Andersen, O. P., Hansen, P. & Madsen, H. (1981). Hyperprolactinaemic amenorrhea induced by metoclopramide. *Acta Obstetrica et Gynecologica Scandinavica*, 60, 341–2.

Bain, S. C., Lemon, M. & Jones, A. F. (1990). Gemfibrozil-induced impotence. *Lancet*, 336, 1389.

Berlin, R. G. (1986). Metoclopramide-induced reversible impotence. *Western Journal of Medicine*, 144, 359–61.

Bharani, A. (1992). Sexual dysfunction after gemfibrizol. *British Medical Journal*, 305, 693.

Bremner, W. J. & Paulsen, C. A. (1976). Colchicine and testicular function in man. *New England Journal of Medicine*, 294, 1384–5.

Briggs, M. H. (1973a). Vitamin C and infertility. *Lancet*, ii, 677–8.

Briggs, M. H. (1973b). Fertility and high-dose vitamin C. *Lancet*, ii, 1083.

Coleman, R. & MacDonald, D. (1994). Effects of isotretinoin on male reproductive system. *Lancet*, 344, 198.

Dutertre, J. P., Soutif, D., Jonville, A. P., Cadenne, M., Valat, J. P. & Autret, E. (1991). Sexual disturbance during omeprazole therapy. 1991, *Lancet*, 338, 1022.

Ehrenfeld, M., Brzezinski, A., Levy, M. & Eliakim, M. (1987). Fertility and obstetric history in patients with familial mediterranean fever on long-term colchicine therapy. *British Journal of Obstetrics and Gynaecology*, 94, 1186–91.

Ehrenfeld, M., Levy, M., Margolith, E. J. & Eliakim, M. (1986). The effect of long term colchicine therapy on male fertility in patients with familial mediterranean fever. *Andrologia*, 18, 420–6.

Epstein, R. J., Allen, R. C. & Lunde, M. W. (1987). Organic impotence associated with carbonic anhydrase inhibitor therapy for glaucoma. *Annals of Ophthalmology*, 19, 48–50.

Evans, B. E. & Aledort, L. M. (1978). Inhibition of ejaculation due to epsilon aminocaproic acid. *New England Journal of Medicine*, 298, 166–7.

Falaschi, P., Frajese, G., Sciarra, F., Rocco, A. & Conti, C. (1978). Influence of hyperprolactinaemia due to metoclopramide on gonadal function in men. *Clinical Endocrinology*, 8, 427–33.

Figueras, A., Castel, M. A., Laporte, J. -R. & Capellà, D. (1993). Gemfibrozil-induced impotence. *Annals of Pharmacotherapy*, 27, 982.

Halkier-Sørensen, L. (1987). Menstrual changes in a patient treated with etretinate. *Lancet*, ii, 636.

Heger, J. J., Solow, E. B., Prystowsky, E. N. & Zipes, D.P. (1984). Plasma and red blood cell concentrations of amiodarone during chronic therapy. *American Journal of Cardiology*, 53, 912–17.

Hilderbrand, R. D. & Hepperlen, T. W. (1990). Lovastatin and hypospermia. *Annals of Internal Medicine*, 112, 549–50.

Hoffer, A. (1973). Vitamin C and infertility. *Lancet*, ii, 1146.

Kennedy, S. H., Forman, R. G., & Barlow, D. H. (1991). Non-steroidal anti–inflammatory drugs and infertility. *Journal of Obstetrics and Gynaecology*, 11, 151–2.

Killick, S. & Elstein, M. (1987). Pharmacological production of luteinized unruptured follicles by prostaglandin synthetase inhibitors. *Fertility and Sterility*, 47, 773–7.

Lardinois, C. K. & Mazzaferri, E. L. (1985). Cimetidine blocks testosterone synthesis. *Archives of Internal Medicine*, 145, 920–2.

Lindquist, M. & Edwards, I. R. (1992). Endocrine adverse effects of omeprazole. *British Medical Journal*, 305, 451–2.

McHaffie, D. J., Guz, A. & Johnston, A. (1977). Impotence in patient on disopyramide. *Lancet*, i, 859.

Merlin, H. E. (1972). Azoospermia caused by colchicine. A case report. *Fertility and Sterility*, 23, 180–1.

Miller, L. G., Rogers, J. C. & Swee, D. E. (1989). Indomethacin-associated sexual dysfunction. *Journal of Family Practice*, 29, 210–11.

Mori, K., Kaido, M., Fujishoro, K. & Inoue, N. (1989). Testicular damage induced by megadoses of pyridoxine. *Sangyo Ika Daigaku Zasshi*, 11, 455–9.

Neri, A., Zukerman, Z., Aygen, M., Lidor, Y. & Kaufournalman, H. (1987). The effect of long term administration of digoxin on plasma androgens and sexual dysfunction. *Journal of Sex and Marital Therapy*, 13, 58–63.

Parsch, E.-M., Ruzucka, Th., Przybilla, B. & Schill, W.-B. (1989). Andrological investigations in men treated with acitretin (Ro 10–1670). *Andrologia*, 22, 479–82.

Peden, N. R., Cargill, J. M., Browning, M. C. K., Saunders, J. H. B. & Wormsley, K. G. (1979). Male sexual dysfunction during treatment with cimetidine. *British Medical Journal*, 1, 659.

Peden, N. R. & Wormsley, K. G. (1982). Effect of cimetidine on gonadal function in man. *British Journal of Clinical Pharmacology*, 14, 565.

Peden, N. R. & Wormsley, K. G. (1983). Alleged impotence with ranitidine. *Lancet*, ii, 798.

Pierce, J. R. Jr. (1983). Cimetidine-associated depression and loss of libido in a woman. *American Journal of the Medical Science*, 286, 31–4.

Reynolds, O. D. (1991). Erectile dysfunction in etretinate treatment. *Archives of Dermatology*, 127, 425–6.

Schneider, J. & Kaffarnik, H. (1975). Impotence in patients treated with clofibrate. *Atherosclerosis*, 21, 455–7.

Van Thiel, D. H., Gavaler, J. S., Smith, W. I. Jr & Paul, G. (1979). Hypothalamic–pituitary–gonadal dysfunction in men using cimetidine. *New England Journal of Medicine*, 300, 1012–5.

Wallace, T. R., Fraunfelder, F. T., Petursson, G. J. & Epstein, D. L. (1979). Decreased libido – a side effect of carbonic anhydrase inhibitor. *Annals of Ophthalmology*, 11, 1563–6.

Wang, C., Wong, K. L., Lam, K. C. & Lai, C. L. (1983). Ranitidine does not affect gonadal function in man. *British Journal of Clinical Pharmacology*, 16, 430–2.

Wei, N. & Hood, J. C. (1980). Naproxen and ejaculatory dysfunction. *Annals of Internal Medicine*, 93, 933.

White, M. C., Gore, M. & Jewell, D. P. (1979). Endocrine function after cimetidine. *New England Journal of Medicine*, 301, 501.

Wolfe, M. M. (1979). Impotence on cimetidine treatment. *New England Journal of Medicine*, 300, 94.

Zorgniotti, A. W., Rossman, B. & Claire, M. (1987). Possible role of chronic use of nasal vasoconstrictors in impotence. *Urology*, 30, 594.

8

Recreational drugs and drugs of abuse

Tobacco

Tobacco is the most significant reproductive poison in current use. It is estimated that each year in North America there are 100 000 fetal deaths, 5000 congenital malformations and 200 000 babies who are born growth retarded as a consequence of maternal cigarette smoking (Hughes, 1994). Given this enormous effect on pregnancy outcome, it would be surprising if smoking did not also have some influence on the ability to conceive. However, despite the huge number of smokers it has proved impossible to reach definitive conclusions of the influence of smoking on conception. There are several reasons for this.

Smoking is more likely to be associated with other factors that can influence fertility, such as pelvic infection and the use of alcohol and caffeine. Small retrospective trials are of inadequate statistical power to reach valid conclusions and only a few large prospective studies have been performed. The design of the studies may introduce bias. One, for example, investigating the effect of smoking on sperm count, selected smokers from an infertility clinic whereas non-smoking controls were selected from men of proved fertility (Vine *et al.*, 1994).

Studies have concentrated on the effects of smoking by men on their sperm parameters, on the chances of conception in women smokers and, more recently, on the influence of smoking on the results of *in vitro* fertilisation. These areas will be reviewed separately.

Effects on sperm

Several reports mention negative effects of nicotine on sperm. One investigation in fertility clinic patients reported that 41% of smokers had reduced sperm density compared with 26% of non-smokers. There was also a reduction in sperm motility in 35% of smokers and 26% of non-smokers (Campbell & Harrison, 1979).

Another study found a greater percentage of abnormal sperm forms in men attending an infertility clinic who were smokers, although no relation could be established between the number of cigarettes smoked and the degree of abnormality (Evans & Fletcher, 1981). There were 42% abnormal forms in 43 non-smokers compared with 47% abnormal forms in the cigarette smokers. They hypothesised that the increase abnormality rate could reflect genetic damage to sperm cells.

Sperm quality in another study of 253 men attending an infertility clinic showed that sperm density and motility were significantly decreased in the smoker group compared with non-smokers. In the smokers group, 75% showed a sperm density of less than 40×10^6 sperm/ml compared with 26% in the non-smoker group. Although morphologic abnormalities were more often prevalent in smokers, no significant difference was found between groups (Kulikauskas, Blaustein & Ablin, 1985).

Sperm abnormalities have also been found in a population of volunteer men. No difference was found in sperm morphology but sperm motility was found to decrease more rapidly in the smoker group. The volume of semen was less in heavy smokers (Saaranen *et al.*, 1987).

A placebo-controlled trial has suggested that the sperm quality of heavy smokers could be improved by supplementation with vitamin C at a dose above 200 mg/day (Dawson *et al.*, 1992).

Motility of sperm has been measured objectively using a laser Doppler technique to measure light reflected from moving sperm. Oldereid *et al.* (1989) studied 350 men from a fertility clinic, who were divided into three groups according to the number of cigarettes smoked per day. No differences were found between smokers and non-smokers for sperm density or motility. Similarly many other studies have not demonstrated any adverse effect of smoking on sperm parameters (Osser, Beckman-Ramirez & Liedholm, 1992; Dunphy *et al.*, 1991).

A most useful contribution to this debate has recently been published by Vine *et al.* (1994). These authors performed a meta-analysis of all papers published between 1966 and 1992 that had addressed sperm density in smokers compared with non-smokers. They excluded papers with obvious selection bias, as described earlier. A total of 20 different study populations were available for analysis, which included 2145 smokers and 2655 controls. The studies were broken down into those performed in men from fertility clinics and those in normal male volunteers. The overall result of the meta-analysis was that the sperm density in smokers was on average between 13 to 17% lower than that of non-smokers. Interestingly, the smoking-related reduction of sperm density in normal men is greater than that seen in infertile patients. These results are probably the most valid published to date on the influence of smoking on sperm concentration.

Effect on fertility

There have only been two large prospective studies looking at the chances of conception in couples in which the female partner is a smoker. The largest study to date included 4104 women who stopped using contraception in order to try to conceive. Howe *et al.* (1985) found a consistent trend of decreasing fertility with an increase in the number of cigarettes smoked a day. Eighteen months after stopping contraception, 28% of heavy smokers had not had a baby in comparison to 19% of non-smokers; after 36 months the difference remained, respectively, 14.2% and 7.8%. After 5 years, 11% of smokers and 5% of non-smokers had not delivered. There was a dose-response relationship between the number of cigarettes smoked per day and fertility. Women who were ex-smokers did not show any evidence of decreased fertility. No increase in the incidence of miscarriages was seen in the smokers.

The only other prospective epidemiological study was published in 1988 and came to the opposite conclusion. A French group studied 1887 couples who were trying to conceive (De Mouzon, Spira & Schwartz, 1988). When crude conception rates were considered at the end of 1 year, 85% of non-smoking women had conceived compared with 70% of smokers. However when all the confounding variables were included in the analysis, smoking was no longer linked to the occurrence of pregnancy. The authors pointed out that one of the significant differences between this study and the study by Howe *et al.* (1985) was that only 68 women in the present study smoked more than 15 cigarettes per day whereas the study by Howe and co-workers only showed a significant decrease in fertility for women smoking more than this.

Retrospective studies are more numerous. In a study performed in 1069 infertile couples and 4305 fertile controls, a significant trend was observed between smoking habit and conception delay. Women smokers showed a risk of delayed conception twice as long as non-smoker women (Olsen *et al.*, 1983).

Baird and Wilcox (1985) found that smokers were 3.4 times more likely to take more than a year to conceive than non-smokers. Fertility of women smokers was estimated to be 72% of the fertility of non-smokers and in each cycle smokers had only 67% as much chance of conceiving as non-smokers. Fertility of heavy smokers fell to 57% of that of non-smokers. Thirty one women who stopped smoking a year before trying to conceive showed no difference in fertility compared with women who had never smoked. Although this is a small sample, this trend is similar to results found in other studies. An analysis of all retrospective studies published showed an overall decreased chance of conception. The chance of pregnancy in smokers in these studies is between 33% and 100% that of non-smokers. Of the nine prospective and retrospective studies that have been published only one, that of De Mouzon *et al.* (1988), has failed to show a negative effect of smoking on fertility (Hughes, 1994).

Effects on in vitro *fertilisation*

Recently it has been possible to examine the influence of cigarettes on fertility more directly by examining subtle end points of the fertilisation process during assisted conception procedures. Evidence exists to suggest that cigarettes may have a direct ovarian effect as smoking is associated with an earlier menopause. Also, products of cigarette smoke have been shown to inhibit the granulosa cell enzyme system that is responsible for converting androgens to oestrogens in the ovary. One recent study showed that smokers undergoing *in vitro* fertilisation developed fewer follicles and had fewer eggs retrieved than non-smokers. This was associated with lower oestrogen levels in blood. There was a raised ratio of androgens to oestrogens in follicular fluid, compatible with an inhibitory effect of cigarette smoking on ovarian granulosa cell enzymes (Van Voorhis *et al.*, 1992). In an *in vitro* study performed by Rosevear *et al.* (1992) conitine, a metabolite of nicotine, was measured in follicular fluid and correlated with oocyte fertilisation rate: 72% of oocytes originating from follicles with a low conitine concentration fertilised compared with 44% in oocytes from follicles with a high conitine concentration.

Impotence

Cigarette smoking is a known risk factor for atherosclerosis. This tendency to atherosclerosis appears to include the arteries supplying the penis. The risk of impotence caused by atherosclerotic disease of the internal pudendal artery was a third higher in smokers than in non-smokers. Smoking also seemed to increase the tendency to form cavernous artery atherosclerosis following chronic perineal trauma (Rosen et al., 1991).

Alcohol

The effects of alcohol on reproductive function can be divided into those that result from acute alcohol consumption by otherwise healthy individuals (social drinking) and those secondary to chronic alcoholism. The latter effects are not just caused by the pharmacological effects of ethanol but are compounded by secondary systemic disturbances induced by alcohol, including liver disease, malnutrition and domestic disharmony. Furthermore, a significant proportion of female alcoholics in one study had a history of sexual dysfunction before becoming alcoholics (McWaine & Procci, 1988). This demonstrates the difficulty in trying to establish cause and effect in this situation.

The effects of alcohol consumption were well known to Shakespeare, who commented in Macbeth that alcohol 'provokes the desire but takes away the performance' Shakespeare's observations were based on anecdotal evidence but have been confirmed in the more rigorous laboratory setting. In one study, 60% of male and 65% of female alcohol abusers found their sexual function improved by alcohol (Smith, Wesson & Apter-Marsh, 1984). Studies have been performed in which alcohol is administered to men and women who are exposed to visual or auditory erotic material. Penile erection and vaginal vasocongestion were measured. Alcohol increased the subjective impression of sexual arousal but reduced the objectively measured signs (Wilson, Niaura & Adler, 1985; Buffum, 1982). Alcohol also causes orgasmic delay in women (Wilson & Lawson, 1976).

Alcohol depresses testosterone concentrations in men following acute ingestion. The low testosterone is associated with a subsequent rise in LH concentration, suggesting a direct toxic effect on the testis (Mendleson, Mello & Ellingboe, 1977; Bertello *et al.,* 1986). Testosterone rises again as the blood alcohol level falls. In contrast, in women, acute alcohol intoxication has no effect on LH or oestrogen levels (Mendleson, Mello & Ellingboe, 1981) although menstrual disturbances and anovulatory cycles have been reported. A large national survey in the USA in 1981 correlated drinking behaviour and reproductive function in a representative sample of 917 women. Dysmenorrhoea, menorrhagia and premenstrual pain were related to the alcohol consumption and were strongly associated with drinking more than six drinks a day at least once per week. Also women consuming six drinks per day at least five times a week had higher levels of infertility (Wilsnack, Klassen & Wilsnack, 1984). The survey does not exclude the possibility that the women drank alcohol because of their gynaecological disorder.

Testosterone concentrations are supressed in chronic alcoholics both in the presence and in the absence of liver disease. Alcohol-induced liver disease alters metabolic processes so that androgens are metabolised to oestrogens. This may lead to gynaecomastia. The combination of low testosterone and high oestrogen is also associated with other signs of feminisation and impotence seen in alcoholics. In one study, 7% of impotent men attending an outpatient clinic were alcoholic (Slag *et al.,* 1983). Similarly in a study of 17000 alcoholic patients, 8% were impotent (Lemere & Smith, 1973). Low testosterone levels are also associated with decreased spermatogenesis leading to oligozoospermia.

In chronic alcoholics, the sexual dysfunction is related to the quantity, frequency and duration of drinking. One study showed that 59% of men attending an alcoholism programme experienced problems with erection and 48% difficulties with ejaculation during bouts of heavy drinking (Mandell & Miller, 1983). Chronic alcoholism may result in permanent impotence even after the complete cessation of drinking for many years (Smith & Asch, 1987).

An assessment of men from infertile couples showed that a group of heavy alcohol consumers had an increase in the number of inflammatory cells in semen (Close, Roberts & Berger, 1990). The authors suggested that the presence of pyospermia may indicate an inflammatory response resulting from testicular damage. Another recent study in 225 infertile men found that regular alcohol consumption was associated with poor results at postcoital testing where sperm numbers and movement are assessed in the females cervical mucus following sexual intercourse (Gerhard *et al.,* 1992).

Marijuana

The fact that marijuana affects sexual function has been known since time immemorial. However despite numerous studies performed over the past few decades, the nature of the sexual effects are still not understood. It was used as an aphrodisiac in ancient Roman and Arabic cultures, while Pliny warned of its tendency to cause impotence. Indian ascetics also used marijuana to 'destroy sexual appetite' (Abel, 1981). It is also difficult to review the literature on this subject without being aware of the potential for subconscious bias on the part of the study investigators. It will come as no surprise to learn that studies supported by grants from the National Institute on Drug Abuse tend to present marijuana in a less favourable light than those from free medical clinics in the San Francisco area.

The main area of investigation concerning the sexual effects of marijuana focus on its effect on libido, sex hormones, sperm parameters and, latterly, fertility.

Effect on libido

Several questionnaire-based studies on this topic have been well reviewed by Abel (1981). There is an association between the degree of marijuana use and measures of sexual activity such as an increased frequency of pre-marital sex and the number of sexual partners. However there is no direct evidence linking drug use to sexual activity and a plausible hypothesis would be that people who have a wish to experiment with sex are also prepared to experiment with drugs. Many respondents to questionnaires reported that one marijuana cigarette increased sexual desire while two or more decreased sexual enjoyment, suggesting a dose-related effect on libido. Abel suggests that the environmental circumstances are more important at low doses whereas the pharmacological effects of drug use predominate at higher doses. No data are offered, however, to support this contention.

Effect on sex hormones

Based on case reports of gynaecomastia in three men who were long-term consumers of marijuana and an observation that testosterone levels were reduced in a frequent marijuana smoker, Kolodny *et al.* (1974) studied testosterone levels in 20 men who consumed large amounts of the drug. The testosterone levels in users were significantly less than in controls and this was dose related. After a 1 week abstinence from the drug, testosterone levels rose significantly. Heavy users had higher FSH levels than those who consumed less. LH levels were unaffected.

A totally different result was reported in the same year in 27 men who were in a more controlled environment (Mendelson *et al.*, 1974). These volunteers were admitted to a research facility for over a month and issued with dose-standardised marijuana cigarettes. They were closely observed to ensure they did not use any other drugs. This study found no effect of marijuana on testosterone. Several subsequent studies have all also shown no effect. The study by Kolodny *et al.*, (1974) has been criticised on the basis that the subjects were allowed to drink some alcohol and other illicit drug use could not be ruled out, both of which could have been responsible for the reduced testosterone. Also testosterone was sampled on only two occasions in the month, whereas other studies have used daily sampling. A later report from Kolodny demonstrated an acute reduction in testosterone levels 30 minutes after smoking marijuana (see Abel, 1981).

Very few controlled studies have been performed on the effect of marijuana on reproductive hormones in women, presumably related to concerns about any potential teratogenic effect (although no specific defect has been described). In animals tetrahydrocannabinol, the active ingredient of marijuana, has been shown to inhibit LH levels probably through a hypothalamic effect. One study did show that female marijuana users had shorter menstrual cycles than non-smokers (26.8 versus 28.8 days) although there were confounding variables as marijuana users consumed twice as much alcohol as non-users and this is also known to provoke menstrual irregularities. A subsequent placebo-controlled study has shown that a single-dose standardised marijuana cigarette suppressed LH levels by 30% after 1 to 2 hours. This effect, however, was only apparent in the luteal phase. In the follicular phase, there was no difference between marijuana and control (Mendelson *et al.*, 1986). The biological significance of this remains to be explored, although low LH levels could intefere with the function of the corpus luteum and lead to short cycles and potential failure of embryo implantion.

A recent case-controlled epidemiological study raises the possibility for the first time that marijuana use by women may be associated with infertility (Mueller *et al.*, 1990). After adjusting for confounding variables, infertile women were 1.7 times more likely to have used marijuana than fertile controls. The infertility was associated with an ovulation defect, as it was found that women who had smoked marijuana within 1 year of trying to conceive were twice as likely to have infertility linked to ovulation problems compared with women who had never used marijuana. However, the results were not dose dependent, as the chances of ovulation defects were greatest in the infrequent users. The authors commented that this could be explained by response bias, i.e. infertile women tending to report lower use of marijuana because they were unwilling to think that its use could have influenced their fertility. They also commented that animal studies had shown that marijuana disrupted ovulation via a hypothalamic action in a manner that was not dose dependent. This effect was reversible.

Effect on sperm

In the Kolodny study discussed earlier (Kolodny *et al.*, 1974), the mean sperm concentration in those who smoked more than 10 'joints' per week was 27 million/ml, compared with 68 million/ml for those using five to nine 'joints'. However, as only 17 volunteers had a semen analysis performed, the significance of this particular observation is questionable. Studies have been performed in which small numbers of chronic marijuana users were hospitalised and subject to a regimen that involved a 3 to 4 week period of no drug, followed by 4 weeks of smoking marijuana (eight to ten cigarettes per day) followed by a 2 to 4 week non-smoking period. These showed no effect during the smoking period but approximately a 50% reduction in sperm concentration during the subsequent no smoking period. As there was no change in hormone concentrations, these results are compatible with a direct effect of marijuana on the seminiferous tubules (Abel, 1981). The time scale is rather short, however, as spermatogenesis takes approximately 74 days and decreased sperm counts were seen after 4 to 6 weeks with recovery to normal levels within 8 weeks of commencing the smoking period. In the absence of contradictory data, it would be safer to assume that chronic marijuana consumption can decrease sperm concentration.

Cocaine

Cocaine use has reached epidemic proportions in the USA and Europe. Recent estimates from the USA are that 30% of men and 20% of women aged 26 to 34 years have used the drug (Yelian *et al.*, 1994). Cocaine hydrochloride users employ intranasal (snorting) or intravenous routes of administration. It may also be applied topically e.g. to the mucous lining of the mouth, rectum or vagina. Users of freebase cocaine (crack) inhale the vapour obtained by heating the crystals. Sexual effects do not appear to differ between the different routes of administration. General experience is that short-term recreational use is associated with increased sexual performance both in terms of increased libido and delay in orgasm in males. Chronic use is related to impotence in men and anorgasmia in women (Siegel, 1982). One questionnaire-based study in cocaine-addicted patients showed that 65% felt that the drug helped with orgasm and 35% thought that it impaired the ability to ejaculate. In women, only 20% felt that it enhanced sexual desire and orgasmic ability. The remainder believed that it impaired sexual enjoyment (Smith *et al.*, 1984)

Chronic cocaine use is associated with hyperprolactinaemia, although gonadotrophin levels do not seem to be affected (Mendelson *et al.*, 1989). This is probably related to cocaine-induced derangement of the inhibition of prolactin release by dopamine. Galactorrhoea, amenorrhoea and menstrual cycle disturbances have been reported in female cocaine users. These may be secondary to hyperprolactinaemia.

A recent epidemiological study has suggested that cocaine users have 11 times the risk of tubal infertility compared with controls. In fact, the cocaine users in this study were three times more likely than fertile controls to have a history of pelvic inflammatory disease, which is the most common cause of tubal infertility. It would not be appropriate, therefore, to draw the conclusion that the tubal infertility was caused by the cocaine use (Mueller *et al.*,1990). Furthermore only 3 of 84 fertile control patients had used cocaine, and it is difficult to draw meaningful conclusions from such limited data.

Effects on sperm

Recent evidence has also emerged that cocaine use may be associated with poor sperm parameters. Men with low sperm motility were twice as likely to have used cocaine for 5 or more years than men with normal motility. Long-term use was also associated with low concentrations and a high number of abnormal sperm forms. These associations were still valid after adjusting for confounding variables (Bracken *et al.*, 1990).

An *in vitro* study in which sperm were exposed in the laboratory to varying concentrations of cocaine hydrochloride for 15 minutes showed a decrease in certain types of sperm movement (measured using computer-assisted semen analysis) at the highest concentrations tested. In contrast, sperm exposed to cocaine for 2 hours showed no decrease in motility. Cocaine is known to bind rapidly to the sperm membrane with optimal binding occurring at 30 minutes followed by subsequent decreased binding. This could explain the lack of effect on motility after more prolonged sperm exposure to cocaine. There was no effect of cocaine exposure in this study to the results of the zona free hamster egg test (Yelian *et al.*, 1994).

Priapism

A few case reports have described priapism following cocaine administration. In two men the cocaine had been applied to the glans penis to take advantage of its local anaesthetic effects in order to prolong sexual intercourse (Rodríguez-Blázquez, Cardona & Rivera-Herrera, 1990). In another, the route of administration was intranasal (Fiorelli *et al.*, 1990). Hypotheses to explain the priapism include profound penile vasodilatation secondary to stimulation of serotonin release from platelets, or local depletion of noradrenaline preventing detumescence. The latter suggestion is based on the fact that noradrenaline causes contraction of penile arterioles, which reduces bloodflow to the penis.

Caffeine

In 1988, an influential paper focused scientific and media attention on a possible negative effect of caffeine on fertility. In a prospective study, Wilcox and colleagues looked at the chance of having a clinically detectable pregnancy, related to the level of caffeine consumed in beverages (Wilcox, Weinberg & Baird, 1988). One cup of 'real' coffee was estimated to contain 100 mg of caffeine, instant coffee 65 mg, tea 50 mg and cola soft drinks 40 mg. Women who consumed more than 100 mg/day caffeine were classified as having a high caffeine intake. Compared with women drinking less than 100 mg/day, high-caffeine consumers had a 50% reduction in their chance of conception in any particular month. In the low-caffeine group, 6% had not conceived after 12 months. The figure in the high-caffeine group was nearly five times greater at 28%. The risk also appeared to be dose related when the caffeine intake was broken down into five different dose levels. The decreased fertility did not appear to be related to anovulation as detected by hormone measurements. The paper also suggested that the reduction in fertility was related to the recent caffeine intake rather than long-term consumption. The reduction in fertility was still apparent even after adjustment for other variables such as frequency of intercourse and cigarette smoking. The authors were careful to point out the possibility for sources of potential bias in their data and stressed the need for further investigation.

Based on these data, several large retrospective studies were reported with conflicting results. In one series of 6300 women, drinking more than four cups of coffee per day was associated with a reduction in fertility of nearly 50% (Christianson, Oechsli & van den Berg, 1989). Others reported that drinking more than two cups of coffee per day had no association with fertility (Joesoef *et al.*, 1990).

The suggestion has been made that caffeine is not the only potentially harmful agent in coffee, and tannin is present in substantial amounts in coffee, tea and soft drinks. Twelfth century druids had considered tannin to be a most potent cause of sterility (Cramer, 1990). Following on from this suggestion, Wilcox and colleagues reanalysed their original data and found that one caffeinated soft drink per day was associated with a 50%

reduction in the chance of pregnancy and this was greater than would be expected from the caffeine content alone (Wilcox & Weinberg, 1991). They suggested that soft drinks should also be added to the list of agents that should be investigated further.

Two recent studies have added more data to the controversy. An epidemiological study of 1050 women with primary infertility and 3883 women who had recently given birth found that high-caffeine intake (more than two cups of coffee per day) was associated with a 50% increase in the risk of infertility caused by tubal disease or endometriosis (Grodstein *et al.*, 1993). A prospective study in 259 non-medical hospital workers showed no increased fertility risk associated with moderate caffeine intake but a reduction of 40% in women consuming more than two cups per day (Florack, Zielhuis & Rolland, 1994).

Based on all these observations, there is now reasonably strong accumulating evidence that more than two cups of 'real' coffee per day or its equivalent is associated with a halving of the chance of conception. This association is valid even when other factors known to be associated with infertility and coffee consumption (such as smoking) are taken into account. Whether this infertility is caused by caffeine, tannin or some other unidentified factor is as yet unknown.

Heroin and methadone

These drugs will be considered together as they have similar effects on reproductive function and most studies have been performed in patients attending drug addiction programmes and taking these drugs either individually or in combination.

Effects on sexuality

Both heroin and methadone decrease sexual desire and performance in addicts and patients on treatment programmes. It is difficult to establish which of these two drugs has the more profound influence as different studies give conflicting results. The incidence of sexual dysfunction on heroin is up to 90% (Buffum, 1992). However, one of the problems is that, while the dose of methadone administered can be controlled, it is impossible to know the dose of heroin taken by addicts in street preparations. Furthermore, many addicts are taking combinations of drugs. Common sexual problems identified include decreased libido, erectile impotence, ejaculatory failure in men and orgasmic dysfunction in women. Men also report delayed ejaculation, which may be seen by some addicts as beneficial if premature ejaculation has been experienced.

A study of men and women in a methadone maintenance programme showed a negative correlation between the dose of drug and frequency of genital contact and orgasm in women and frequency of ejaculation in men (Crowley & Simpson, 1978). In another programme, 50% of a sample of men in a methadone programme reported sexual dysfunction occurring within 1 month of commencing methadone. It was significant that over two thirds of those who had sexual dysfunction on methadone had also experienced the same problem on heroin, whereas dysfunction on heroin was very rare in men who had no sexual problems on methadone (Hanbury, Cohen & Stimmel, 1977). A recent detailed study of sexual function and psychological profiles of patients stabilised on methadone suggested that disturbed sexual function is more likely to be related to psychiatric problems than to the pharmacological effects of the drug (Spring, Willenbring & Maddux, 1992).

One study attempted to assess semen analyses in addicts and patients on methadone. A third of patients were not able to produce a semen sample as they were unable to ejaculate. These patients were still on heroin. Those on methadone alone were able to provide samples (Ragni *et al.*, 1988).

Effects on hormones

Several studies have demonstrated an effect of opiates on the hypothalamo-pituitary axis. The results are not always in agreement. Some have found decreased LH and low testosterone (Mendelson & Mello, 1982). Others show no change in LH, FSH or testosterone (Cicero *et al.*, 1975; Ragni *et al.*, 1988). Prolactin levels are also variably elevated. One group performing dynamic pituitary testing showed near maximal secretion of prolactin in patients on methadone (Willenbring *et al.*, 1989). Another study showed significant elevations of prolactin on heroin but not on methadone (Ragni *et al.*, 1988). X-ray analysis of the pituitiary fossa were always normal in the hyperprolactinaemic heroin addicts, although this investigation will only detect relatively large pituitary tumours. In another study, prolactin was elevated in methadone-treated patients (Lafisca *et al.*, 1981).

Hormone levels in female heroin addicts have not been included in these studies, but early reports described infrequent and absent periods in two thirds of female heroin addicts. In one methadone maintenance programme, menstruation returned to normal in 82 of 83 women within 1 to 2 months of commencing methadone. It was not possible to say whether this was a drug effect or the result of a return to a more stable environment (Wallach, Jerez & Blinick, 1969).

Effects on sperm

Abnormalities of semen analysis are common in methadone-treated patients. In particular, the volume of ejaculate may be low because of reduced secretions from the prostate and seminal vesicles (Cicero *et al.*, 1975). This early study also showed that ejaculate volume was greater in heroin addicts than in those on methadone. Abnormal sperm parameters were found in 93% of heroin addicts and in 65% of those taking methadone. Poor motility was the most common finding followed by abnormal sperm morphology (Ragni *et al.*, 1985, 1988).

Mechanisms of opiate-induced sexual dysfunction

Several mechanisms have been proposed to account for the varied reproductive adverse effects although the picture is confused because of inconsistency between studies. Some of the dysfunction may be related to lifestyle rather than pharmacology. Severe psychological disturbance, malnutrition and incidental disease are common in addicts. No studies have investigated the recent phenomenon of possible AIDS-related reproductive disturbances in this group. However, the pharmacological effects of opiates may explain some of the problems. Decreased libido could be secondary to reduced plasma testosterone, and erectile dysfunction to opiate-induced cutaneous vasodilatation shunting blood away from the penile vasculature (Buffum, 1982). Heroin also acts as an α-adrenergic blocker, which could interfere with both seminal emission (causing decreased ejaculate volume) and ejaculation (causing retarded ejaculation).

Amphetamines

Amphetamines are central nervous system stimulants and α- and β-adrenergic stimulants. The use of low oral doses of amphetamines is said to stimulate sexual desires while high doses may be associated with impotence and ejaculatory failure in males and anorgasmia in women (Buffum, 1982). Large intravenous doses may provoke orgasm directly. A recent study of intravenous drug abusers included 27 men who had sexual activity while using amphetamines. Twenty three reported that they became more sexually excited on amphetamines and the same number stated that the drug prolonged intercourse. In 21 orgasm was intensified. The authors pointed out that the increased libido of intravenous amphetamine users was a risk factor for transmission of HIV, as only three men had used a condom with their last casual sexual partner (Kall, 1992). The mechanism of ejaculation delay is uncertain but it could be a central action as amphetamine affects many central nervous system transmitters. Alternatively, it has been suggested that it may be caused by increased distractibility reducing coital sensation. The increased intensity of orgasm could be accounted for by α-adrenergic stimulation.

Lysergic acid diethylamide (LSD)

Conflicting effects on sexual function have been attributable to this hallucinogen. Some users describe deeply moving sexual experiences whilst others report a complete absence of sexual feeling. No recent formal studies have been performed.

Amyl nitrites

Commonly referred to as 'poppers', these volatile nitrates have been used as sex enhancers to intensify and prolong orgasm. They act by causing potent vasodilatation but this does sometimes lead to loss of erection probably through peripheral shunting of blood from the penis (McWaine and Procci, 1988).

Ecstasy (methylenedioxymethamphetamine)

Ecstasy is an amphetamine derivative that is a currently popular street drug. It has disinhibiting properties that could enhance libido, although there are no reports of its effects on reproductive function to date.

References

Abel, E. L. (1981). Marihuana and sex: a critical survey. *Drug and Alcohol Dependence*, 8, 1–22.
Baird, D. D & Wilcox, A. J. (1985). Cigarette smoking associated with delayed conception. *Journal of the American Medical Association*, 253, 2979–83.
Bertello, P., Gurioli, L., Gatti, G., Pinna, G. & Angeli, A. (1986) Short term ethanol ingestion can affect the testicular response to single-dose human chorionic gonadotrophin in normal subjects. *Journal of Endocrinological Investigation*, 9, 249–52.
Bracken, M. B., Eskenazi, B., Sachse, K., McSharry, J. E., Hellenbrand, K. &

Leo-Summers, L. (1990). Association of cocaine use with sperm concentration, motility, and morphology. *Fertility and Sterility*, 53, 315–22.

Buffum, J. (1982). Pharmacosexology:the effects of drugs on sexual function. *Journal of Psychoactive Drugs*, 14, 5–44.

Buffum, J. (1992). Prescription drugs and sexual function. *Psychiatric Medicine*, 10, 181–98.

Campbell, J. M. & Harrison, K. L. (1979). Smoking and infertility. *The Medical Journal of Australia*, 1, 342–3.

Christianson, R. E., Oechsli, F. W. & van den Berg, B. J. (1989). Caffeinated beverages and decreased fertility. *Lancet*, i, 378.

Cicero, T. J., Bell, R. D., Wiest, W. G., Allison, J. H., Polakoski, K. & Robins, E. (1975). Function of the male sex organs in heroin and methadone users. *New England Journal of Medicine*, 292, 882–7.

Close, C. E., Roberts, P. L. & Berger, R. E. (1990). Cigarettes, alcohol and marijuana are related to pyospermia in infertile men. *Journal of Urology*, 144, 900–3.

Cramer, D. W. (1990) Letter. *Lancet*, 335, 793.

Crowley, T. J. & Simpson, R. (1978). Methadone dose and human sexual behaviour. *International Journal of the Addictions*, 13, 285–95.

Dawson, E. B., Harris, W. A., Teter, M. C. & Powell, L. C. (1992). Effect of ascorbic acid supplementation on the sperm quality of heavy smokers. *Fertility and Sterility*, 58, 1034–9.

De Mouzon, J., Spira, A. & Schwartz, D. (1988). A prospective study of the relation between smoking and fertility. *International Journal of Epidemiology*, 17, 378–84.

Dunphy, B. C., Barratt, C. L., von Tongelen, B. P. & Cooke, I. D. (1991). Male cigarette smoking and fecundity in couples attending an infertility clinic. *Andrologia*, 23, 223–5.

Evans, H. J. & Fletcher, J. (1981). Sperm abnormalities and cigarette smoking. *Lancet*, i, 627–9.

Fiorelli, R. L., Manfrey, S. J., Belkoff, L. H. & Finkelstein, L. H. (1990). Priapism associated with intranasal cocaine abuse. *Journal of Urology*, 143, 584–5.

Florack, E. I., Zielhuis, G. A. & Rolland, R. (1994). Cigarette smoking, alcohol consumption, and caffeinated intake and fecundability. *Preventative Medicine*, 23, 175–80.

Gerhard, I., Lenhard, K., Eggert-Kruse, W. & Runnebaum, B. (1992). Clinical data which influence semen parameters in infertile men. *Human Reproduction*, 7, 830–7.

Grodstein, F., Goldman, M. B., Ryan, L. & Cramer, D. W. (1993). Relation of female infertility to consumption of caffeinated beverages. *American Journal of Epidemiology*, 137, 1353–60.

Hanbury, R., Cohen, M. & Stimmel, B. (1977). Adequacy of sexual performance in men maintained on methadone. *American Journal of Drug and Alcohol Abuse*, 4, 13–20.

Howe, G., Westhoff, C., Vessey, M. & Yeates, D. (1985). Effects of age, cigarette smoking, and other factors on fertility: findings in a large prospective study. *British Medical Journal*, 290, 1697–1700.

Hughes, E. G. (1994). Smoking and conception. *Orgyn*, v, 24–7.

Joesoef, M. R., Beral, V., Rolfs, R. T., Aral, S. O. & Cramer, D. W. (1990). Are caffeinated beverages risk factors for delayed conception? *Lancet*, 335, 136–7.

Kall, I. (1992). Effects of amphetamine on sexual behaviour of male i. v. drug users in Stockholm – a pilot study. *AIDS Education and Prevention*, 4, 6–17.

Kolodny, R. C., Masters, W. H., Kolodner, R. M. & Toro, G. (1974). Depression of plasma testosterone levels after chronic intensive marihuana use. *New England Journal of Medicine*, 290, 872–4.

Kulikauskas, V., Blaustein, D. & Ablin, R. J. (1985). Cigarette smoking and its possible effects on sperm. *Fertility and Sterility*, 44, 526–8.

Lafisca, S., Bolelli, G., Franceschetti, F., Filicori, M., Flamigni, C. & Marigo, M. (1981). Hormone levels in methadone-treated drug addicts. *Drug and Alcohol Dependence*, 8, 229–34.

Lemere, F. & Smith, J. W. (1973). Alcohol induced sexual impotence. *American Journal of Psychiatry*, 130, 212–13.

Mandell, W. & Miller, C. M. (1983). Male sexual dysfunction as related to alcohol consumption: a pilot study. *Alcoholism, Clinical and Experimental Research*, 7, 65–9.

McWaine, D. E. & Procci, W. R. (1988). Drug-induced sexual dysfunction. *Medical Toxicology*, 3, 289–306.

Mendelson, J. H., Kuehnle, J., Ellingboe, J. & Babor, T. F. (1974). Plasma testosterone levels before, during and after chronic marihuana smoking. *New England Journal of Medicine*, 291, 1051–5.

Mendelson, J. H. & Mello, N. K. (1982). Hormones and psychosexual development in young men following chronic heroin abuse. *Neurobehavioural Toxicology and Teratology*, 4, 441–5.

Mendelson, J. H., Mello, N. K. & Ellingboe, J. (1977). Effects of acute alcohol intake on pituitary gonadal hormones in normal males. *Journal of Pharmacology and Experimental Therapeutics*, 202, 676–82.

Mendelson, J. H., Mello, N. K. & Ellingboe, J. (1981). Acute alcohol intake and pituitary gonadal hormones in normal human females. *Journal of Pharmacology and Experimental Therapeutics*, 218, 23–6.

Mendelson, J. H., Mello, N. K., Ellingboe, J., Skupny, A. S. T., Lex, B. W. & Griffin, M. (1986). Marihuana smoking suppresses luteinising hormone in women. *Journal of Pharmacology and Experimental Therapeutics*, 237, 862–6.

Mendelson, J. H., Mello, N. K., Teoh, S. K., Ellingboe, J. & Cochin, J. (1989). Cocaine effects on pulsatile secretion of anterior pituitary, gonadal, and adrenal hormones. *Journal of Clinical Endocrinology and Metabolism*, 69, 1256–60.

Mueller, B. A., Daling, J. R., Weiss, N. S. & Moore, D. E. (1990). Recreational drug use and the risk of primary infertility. *Epidemiology*, 1, 195–200.

Oldereid, N. B., Rui, H., Clausen, O. P. F. & Purvis, K. (1989). Cigarette smoking and human sperm quality assessed by laser-Doppler spectroscopy and DNA flow cytometry. *Journal of Reproduction and Fertility*, 86, 731–6.

Olsen, J., Rachootin, P., Schiødt, A. V. & Damsbo, N. (1983). Tobacco use, alcohol consumption and infertility. *International Journal of Epidemiology*, 12, 179–84.

Osser, S., Beckman-Ramirez, A. & Liedholm, P. (1992). Semen quality of smoking and non-smoking men in infertile couples in a Swedish population. *Acta Obstetricia Gynecologica Scandinavica*, 71, 215–18.

Ragni, G., De Lauretis, L., Bestetti, O., Sghedoni, D. & Gambaro, V. (1988). Gonadal function in male heroin and methadone addicts. *International Journal of Andrology*, 11, 93–100.

Ragni, G., De Lauretis, L., Gambaro, V., Di Pietro, R, Bestetti, O., Recalcati, F. & Papetti, C. (1985). Semen evaluation in heroin and methadone addicts. *Acta Europaea Fertilitatis*, 16, 245–9.

Rodríguez-Biázquez, H. M., Cardona, P. E. & Rivera-Herrera, J. L. (1990).

Priapism associated with the use of topical cocaine. *Journal of Urology,* 143, 358.

Rosen, M. P., Greenfield, A. J., Walker, T. G., Grant, P., Dubrow, J., Bettmann, M. A., Fried, L. E. & Goldstein, I. (1991). Cigarette smoking: an independent risk factor for atherosclerosis in the hypogastric-cavernous arterial bed of men with arteriogenic impotence. *Journal of Urology*, 145, 759–63.

Rosevear, S. K., Holt, D. W., Lee, T. D., Ford, W. C. L., Wardle, P. G. & Hull, M. G. R. (1992). Smoking and decreased fertilisation rates in vitro. *Lancet*, 340, 1195–6.

Saaranen, M., Suonio, S., Kauhanen, O. & Saarikoski, S. (1987). Cigarette smoking and semen quality in men of reproductive age. *Andrologia*, 19, 670–6.

Siegel, R. K. (1982). Cocaine and sexual dysfunction: the curse of Mama Coca. *Journal of Psychoactive Drugs,* 14, 71–4.

Slag, M. F., Morley, J. E., Elson, M. K., Trence, D. L., Nelson, C. J., Nelson, A. E., Kinlaw, W. B., Beyer, S., Nuttall, F. Q. & Shafer, R. B. (1983). Impotence in medical outpatients. *Journal of the American Medical Association.* 249, 1736–40.

Smith, D.E., Wesson, D. R & Apter-Marsh, W (1984). Cocaine- and alcohol–induced sexual dysfunction in patients with addictive disease. *Journal of Psychoactive Drugs*, 16, 359–61.

Smith, C. G. & Asch, R. H. (1987). Drug abuse and reproduction. *Fertility and Sterility*, 48, 355–73.

Spring, W. D. Jr, Willenbring, M. L. & Maddux, T. L. (1992). Sexual dysfunction and psychological stress in methadone maintenance. *International Journal of the Addictions*, 27, 1325–34.

Van Voorhis, B. J., Syrop, C. H., Hammitt, D. G., Dunn, M. S. & Snyder, G. D. (1992). Effects of smoking on ovulation induction for assisted reproductive techniques. *Fertility and Sterility*, 58, 981–5.

Vine, M. F., Margolin, B. H., Morrison, H. I. & Hulka, B. S. (1994). Cigarette smoking and sperm density: a meta-analysis. *Fertility and Sterility*, 61, 35–43.

Wallach, R. C., Jerez, E. & Blinick, G. (1969). Pregnancy and menstrual function in narcotic addicts treated with methadone. *American Journal of Obstetrics and Gynecology*, 105, 1226–9.

Wilcox, A. J. & Weinberg, C. R. (1991). Tea and fertility. *Lancet,* 337, 1159–60.

Wilcox, A., Weinberg, C. & Baird, D. (1988). Caffeinated beverages and decreased fertility. *Lancet*, ii, 1453–6.

Willenbring, M. L., Morley, J. E., Krahn, D. D., Carlson, G. A., Levine, A. S. & Shafer, R. B. (1989). Psychoneuroendocrine effects of methadone maintenance. *Psychoneuroendocrinology*, 14, 371–91.

Wilsnack, S. C., Klassen A. D. & Wilsnack, R. W. (1984). Drinking and reproductive dysfunction among women in a 1981 national survey. *Alcoholism, Clinical and Experimental Research*, 8, 541–8.

Wilson, G. T. & Lawson, D. (1976). Effects of alcohol on sexual arousal in women. *Journal of Abnormal Psychology*, 85, 489–97.

Wilson, G. T., Niaura, R. S. and Adler J. L. (1985). Alcohol, selective attention and sexual arousal in men. *Journal of Studies on Alcohol*, 46, 107–15.

Yelian, F. D., Sacco, A. G., Ginsburg, K. A., Doerr, P. A. & Armant, D. R. (1994). The effects of in vitro cocaine exposure on human sperm motility, intracellular calcium, and ooctye penetration. *Fertility and Sterility*, 61, 915–21.

9

Fertility and the environment

Introduction

We live, work, eat and breathe in an environment filled with agents that have the potential for reproductive toxicity. There are over 60 000 chemicals in use in manufacturing processes and over 500 are added each year. Men and women can be exposed to these agents if they work in manufacturing industries producing or utilising the products; however, we all consume and accumulate chemicals because of our position as the terminal link in the food chain. We drink contaminated water. We are in contact with toxic chemicals when we decorate our houses and indulge in our hobbies. We are surrounded by sources of ionising and non-ionising radiation. In short it is impossible to avoid exposure to potential reproductive toxicants.

Certain environmental agents (comparatively few) have been proved by rigorous experimentation to have a major deleterious effect on reproductive performance. Many more have been linked to reproductive dysfunction but hard proof is lacking. It is highly likely that several environmental toxicants have as yet undiscovered adverse effects. Furthermore, we are exposed daily to low levels of toxicants, lead and radiation for example, which are known to have serious adverse effects on reproductive functions above certain threshold levels. Maximum permitted exposure levels have been calculated, but it is impossible to predict a level that is not harmful.

Reproductive toxicology is a very new branch of occupational medicine. The first significant report describing the effect of the pesticide dibromochloropropane (DBCP) was only published in 1977. There is now much more consumer interest in environmental issues in general and the importance of toxicants as a cause of infertility is starting to create deep concern in both lay and scientific communities.

Types of reproductive dysfunction

Chemicals can interfere with fertility by acting at virtually any of the sites that control sexual function. In men, toxicants have been shown to have a number of effects: altering hormone concentrations and hormone metabolism (lead and dichlorodiphenyltrichloroethane (DDT)); interfering with Leydig cells (DBCP); disrupting spermatogenesis (DBCP); and reducing seminal plasma volume (ethylene dibromide, (EDB)) (Schrader and Kesner 1994). In women, adverse effects have been found in hypothalamic pituitary function (lead, DDT, polychlorinated biphenyls (PCB), polybrominated biphenyls (PBB)); granulosa cells (mercury); and ovarian follicles (polycyclic aromatic hydrocarbons, cadmium) (Plowchalk, Meadows & Mattison, 1994).

Infertility is only one part of the spectrum of reproductive disorders caused by environmental toxicants. Other effects include early and late miscarriage, congenital abnormality, premature delivery, low birth weight and stillbirth. Sexual dysfunction and premature menopause can also develop. Although these may all result in the inability to have normal healthy children, the scope of this chapter will be limited to those effects resulting in inability to conceive and not the inability to carry a normal pregnancy through to a live delivery.

Assessment of reproductive dysfunction

Some toxicants have a rapid and marked effect that is easily noted, for example irradiation leading to ovarian failure and a premature menopause. However, the effect is often more subtle and may only be discovered following detailed investigation. Several methods are available to assess fertility in the context of exposure to toxicants (Baranski, 1993).

Number of pregnancies in a lifetime

The best way to prove that fertility is reduced is to assess the total number of children born to couples in whom one or both partners may have been exposed. As a typical family may have two children over a lifetime, generations may need to elapse before a meaningful result can be calculated. This measure is also subject to many of the confounding variables described later.

Time to first pregnancy

An alternative measure is the time to first pregnancy, based on the assumption that in a typical fertile couple the woman has a 1 in 5 chance of falling pregnant each month. This is quite an accurate technique if performed prospectively, although if retrospective, memory recall bias will be a problem. It can also only be applied to couples who conceive; therefore, potentially the most severely affected cases, those whose exposure has rendered them infertile, will be excluded from this analysis.

Infertility rate

The infertility rate can be defined as the inability to produce a clinically recognisable pregnancy after 1 year of unprotected intercourse. This also requires large populations and is a relatively insensitive measurement. Furthermore, it excludes recurrent embryonic loss before the stage of clinically detectable pregnancy. As a working definition though it is practical.

Measurement of expected to observed live births

Figures are available to predict the expected number of births for a given population taking into account, age, parity, racial group, etc. This can be compared with the actual number in an exposed population. This ratio can only be used for large studies and will exclude any adverse reproductive outcome not associated with a live birth i.e. miscarriage.

Confounding variables

There are many confounding variables to any measure of fertility. The major ones include other non-associated infertility factors, such as the presence of sexually transmitted disease in either partner, frequency of intercourse, stability of the couple's relationship as well as lifestyle factors, age, etc. Most of these points can be addressed by carefully controlled studies.

Indirect measures of fertility

The most common method of assessing male fertility for toxicological studies is semen analysis, although results are variable both within and between individuals. Also attempts to correlate sperm counts etc. to fertility have shown that it is a measure of limited value. Sperm count, movement (motility) and normality (morphology) are quantified. Sperm viability can also be assessed as a sperm that is not moving is not necessarily dead. The volume of seminal plasma is measured and biochemical analysis of seminal fluid performed to investigate accessory gland function. Reproductive hormone concentrations (FSH, LH, testosterone) and binding proteins (sex hormone-binding globulin) can also be measured in blood.

More recently introduced techniques in reproductive toxicology include computer-assisted semen analysis, zona-free hamster egg penetration tests, which measure the fertilising potential of human sperm in hamster eggs, and the DNA stability test, which seems to be a highly reproducible assay for sperm DNA damage (Scialli, 1992).

In females, indirect measures of fertility include reproductive hormone measurements and menstrual calendars, which note cycle length and regularity. Newer tests include the *in vitro* culture of ovarian granulosa cells to test the steroidogenic potential of these cells. In patients having infertility treatment, the ability of the eggs to be fertilised and form embryos can be assessed using *in vitro* fertilisation techniques.

Animal tests

Animal studies using rodents in particular have established the potential reproductive toxicity as well as mechanisms of action of many environmental agents. The results, however, are frequently not applicable to humans because of differences in reproductive physiology and metabolism.

Mode of action of reproductive toxicants

Reproductive toxicants can be divided into two categories based on their modes of action (Mattison and Thomford 1989; Plowchalk *et al.*, 1994).

Direct-acting toxicants

Direct-acting toxic agents affect reproduction either through their chemical reactivity or by their structural similarity to an endogenous substance. Chemically reactive toxicants damage important cellular components and tend to be non-specific, for example alkylating agents used in cancer chemotherapy. Lead, mercury and cadmium also probably act in this way.

Structurally similar toxicants confuse the body into believing that they are biologically important compounds, for example hormones. Many are hormone agonists or antagonists. The classical example here would be the combined contraceptive pill. It has been shown that occupational exposure to synthetic oestrogens and progestogens has led to infertility by suppression of gonadotrophin levels. Other toxicants with oestrogenic activity include PCB and PBB and organochlorine pesticides.

Toxicants acting indirectly

Indirect toxicants alter normal processes in one of two ways. They can be metabolised to a product that is more toxic than the parent compound or they can act by modifying naturally occurring enzymes or hormones.

Enzymes present within the ovary and testis are responsible for the metabolic processing of many compounds that result in reproductive toxicity, for example cyclophosphamide, polycyclic aromatic hydrocarbons (PAH) and DBCP.

Other reproductive toxicants induce or inhibit enzymes in the gonads and liver that are involved in hormone metabolism. By interfering with hormone feedback pathways, normal reproductive control can be lost. Examples in this category include DDT, PCB and PBB.

Sources of toxicant exposure

There are three ways of becoming exposed to environmental reproductive toxicants.

> **Acute poisoning.** This typically affects workers in an industrial facility or people living in close proximity to a plant when an accident causes the release of high levels of toxicant.
>
> **Chronic occupational exposure.** This is caused by long-term exposure to ambient levels of toxicant within the workplace environment.
>
> **Environmental exposure.** All plants, animals and humans are now exposed to toxicants in their air, water and food.

Most information on reproductive hazards has arisen as a consequence of the first two mechanisms of exposure, which usually involves contamination levels much higher than those occurring within the natural environment. However, very little information is available about levels found in the environment, which, until recently, were not thought to pose a threat to reproduction. It is a measure of the concern currently felt by the public that governmental organisations charged with environmental safety are now starting to give as much weight to the reproductive dangers of environmental agents as to their carcinogenic potential.

The rest of this chapter will discuss toxicants that have been proved to have, or are strongly suspected of having, a negative impact on fertility or sexual function. Much information has been obtained from an excellent book published recently to which readers with a particular interest in this topic are referred (Paul, 1994a).

Radiation

Ionising radiation

Measurements of ionising radiation

Ionising radiation can be produced by electromagnetic waves (X-rays and gamma rays) and charged particles (α and β particles). The number of ionisations produced by radiation in air is measured in röntgens (R). Of more clinical relevance is the rad (*radiation absorbed dose*), which is a measure of the energy absorbed during the interaction of the radiation within the tissue. Depending on the type of ionising radiation the same energy absorbed can produce different degrees of biological damage. For example α particles produce 20 times the biological damage of gamma rays and X-rays. The absorbed dose is therefore multiplied by a 'radiation weighting factor' to give the *equivalent dose*. Finally, different tissues of the body have different radiosensitivities. The gonads, for example are much more sensitive than the surface of the bones. The equivalent dose is, therefore, multiplied by a 'tissue weighting factor' to take into account the overall risk of any combination of radiation affecting any or all the tissues in the body. This is referred to as the *effective dose* and is the standard measure of human exposure to radiation. It is measured in sievert (Sv) units. Millisieverts (mSv) and microsieverts (μSv) are usually employed to describe the doses received by humans (National Radiation Protection Board, 1994).

Exposure levels

Everyone is exposed to ionising radiation. In the USA, the annual effective dose for the average person is 3 mSv. The latest available figures for the UK are from 1991 (Hughes, 1993). The average annual effective dose is 2.6 mSv. This is made up of natural exposures and artificial exposures. Natural exposures account for 2.2 mSv (85%) of which 1.3 mSv is from radon (a natural inert gas produced by the spontaneous radioactive decay of uranium 238 found in the earth's crust). This depends on geographical location (it can be 100 times greater in certain counties) and workplace environment. Coal miners are particularly exposed. Cosmic radiation accounts for 250 μSv but this increases with altitude, particularly during airline travel. Aircrew, for example, receive an annual dose of nearly 1000 times this value. Other sources of natural exposure are in food and drink (300 μSv) and gamma rays (350 μSv)

The main route of artificial exposure is through medical X-rays (370 μSv). Small amounts of exposure result from radioactive fallout from past atmospheric weapons tests (5 μSv) and discharge of radioactive effluent (0.5 μSv). Similarly low exposure occurs from consumer products such as luminous watches and smoke alarms (0.4 μSv). The main occupational exposure occurs in workers in the nuclear industry. The average dose received was 0.5 mSv although 10 workers in 1991 received greater than 15 mSv. In 1987, 1100 workers received a dose in excess of 15 mSv.

The present annual legal dose limit is 50 mSv per year, although the National Radiation Protection Board recommends a dose limit for workers of 20 mSv. This level of exposure would correspond to an annual risk of fatal cancer of 1/1000 (National Radiation Protection Board, 1994).

There are three principle sources of information on reproductive injury induced by ionising radiation: patients having therapeutic irradiation, survivors of nuclear explosions and prisoners subject to testicular irradiation. Some important concepts determine reproductive effects of ionising radiation (Brent, Meistrich & Paul, 1994). These include speed of cell division, fractionation of radiation dose and age of the exposed individual. These will be discussed separately for each sex.

Ionising radiation in men

Speed of cell division. Rapidly dividing cells are the most radiosensitive and this has important clinical implications. The differentiating spermatogonia are the most radiosensitive whereas spermatids do not divide and are relatively radioresistant. Similarly Leydig and Sertoli cells are usually unaffected by moderate radiation doses. Following testicular irradiation, there are four phases in sperm response.

For the first 2 months after irradiation, there is relatively little effect on sperm count as the more mature spermatids and spermatozoa continue to be ejaculated. In the second phase, there is a significant reduction in the sperm count. The magnitiude of the reduction depends on the testicular dose. After a dose of less than 20 rad, few men become azoospermic whereas after 100 rad 90% develop azoospermia. In the third phase, recovery of sperm production can occur, which may be followed by recovery to normal levels in the final phase. Reductions in normal morphology and motility accompany the changes in sperm count.

Fractionation of dose. It is a general principle of radiobiology that tissues recover more following multiple small doses than from a single large dose as the damaged tissues are able to repair themselves. Unfortunately for the testis, the reverse is true as the stem cell response to irradiation is to proliferate, which makes it more radiosensitive to the next dose of radiation. Therefore 2 years following a single dose of less than 600 rad, nearly all azoospermic men will have recovered sperm production. If a dose of greater than 200 rad is given in fractionated doses, 85% will remain azoospermic after 2 years.

Ionising radiation in women

The principles that apply to men apply equally to women. As the great majority of oocytes are within non-dividing primary follicles, the ovary is relatively resistant to ionising radiation compared with the testicle. Doses of less than 60 rad appear to have no effect. Atomic bomb survivors in Japan exposed to doses exceeding 100 rad had no reductions in fertility. However, because of the reducing pool of ovarian follicles with age, the effect of ovarian irradiation increases with age. Permanent sterility was induced by ovarian irradiation (250–500 rad) in the majority of women over the age of 40, whereas younger women only experienced transient menstrual disturbances.

The dose of X-rays in diagnostic procedures is very low compared with the values above. For example a women would need 30 000 chest X-rays or 120 hysterosalpingograms to receive a dose of 60 rad.

Non-ionising radiation

Radio-frequency radiation including microwave radiation as well as radiation produced in electromagnetic fields fall into this category. Tissue damage is caused, not by the production of ions but by heat generation, which depends on several factors including the wavelength of the radiation (Brent, *et al.,* 1994). Long wavelength radiation produced by electric power cables, for example, can pass through the body without giving up energy in the form of heat. High frequency (short) wavelengths such as those used in microwave ovens produce considerable heat within tissue. There is much public concern regarding the potential health risks of electromagnetic radiation, although there are few data to date on adverse reproductive effects.

Microwave radiation

Only one study has described decreased libido and reduced sperm count, motility and morphology in men who were occupationally exposed to microwaves for a mean time of 8 years. In most cases, this had returned to normal after 3 months.

Magnetic resonance imaging (MRI)

MRI produces both electromagnetic and radiofrequency radiation. There are no studies relating specifically to fertility aspects of low-frequency electromagnetic fields. Radiofrequency radiation is known to increase tissue temperature but the energies used in MRI have a minimal heating effect. More safety information is obviously needed in this area.

Ultrasound

Ultrasound produces mechanical energy at high frequencies. Although the majority is reflected, which forms the basis for its diagnostic use, some is absorbed. Negligible tissue heating is induced during diagnostic procedures. Two studies have suggested reduced pregnancy rates in women in whom follicular development was being monitored by ultrasound compared with an unmonitored population, although this has been disputed. In therapeutic areas and industrial applications, different ultrasound frequencies are used and tissue heating does occur. This would only be hazardous if there was direct body contact with the material being treated.

Metals

Lead

Sources

An antifertility effect for lead has been suggested since Roman times when the lead content of drinking vessels was suspected to be the cause of declining populations in the upper classes. The spermicidal properties of lead have also been long appreciated (Schragg & Dixon, 1985).

Exposure to lead now is in three forms: occupational exposure, environmental exposure and household use. Occupational exposure occurs, for example, in workers in the smelting industry, in those working with batteries, in stained glass craftsmen and workers in the construction industry, printing, etc. Controls on the use of tetraethyl lead in petrol and other products has reduced environmental exposure but the most common source of lead is within the home. This is in the form of ingestion from contaminated water (contamination occurring from the pipes not the water source), paints and air- and dust-borne contamination. Many hobbies are also associated with significant exposure to lead. These include developing and printmaking, furniture restoration, pottery glazing and electronics.

Mode of action

Lead has antifertility effects in both males and females. One study of 150 men who were heavily exposed reported dose-related reductions in sperm movement and morphology and in semen volume, with no change in gonadotrophin levels. This would be consistent with a direct effect on spermatogenesis and accessory gland function (Schragg & Dixon, 1985). Other studies have noted hormone abnormalities consistent with an effect on the hypothalamo-pituitary-testicular axis. Lead can be found in the testes and semen as well as in the hypothalamus and pituitary. It is possible that acute exposure results in a direct gonadotoxic effect, whereas chronic exposure is associated with hypathalomo-pituitary disturbances. Interestingly, one study has shown that the wives of men whose lead levels were elevated in the year before conception had a higher miscarriage rate (Miller & Bellinger, 1994).

In female rodent studies, postnatal exposure to lead resulted in direct ovarian toxicity as well as decreased FSH, implying a hypothalamo-pituitary effect. Ovarian secretion of progesterone in the luteal phase is also reduced, which may have a negative impact on implantation. Other studies have suggested a direct effect of lead on uterine oestrogen receptors, which may also interfere with implantation (Mattison & Thomford, 1989). In a Danish case control study the time to conception was increased in women exposed to lead (Baranski, 1993).

Mercury

Mercury is found in the environment in two forms. Organic methylmercury is present in high concentration in fish, particularly swordfish, shark and tuna. It is metabolised in the body to inorganic mercury. The principal route of exposure of the general population to inorganic mercury is from dental amalgams. Occupational exposure occurs in mining and manufacturing accidents, as well as in dentists and their assistants.

Long-term exposure, as well as acute poisoning with methylmercury, results in central nervous system damage. Methylmercury has been shown to disrupt spermatogenesis in mice, but there is little information on its effect on human fertility. A dose-dependent reduction in libido was observed in 50 men chronically exposed to methylmercury with no signs of poisoning. They also had defective sperm parameters. Case reports in nine men also described decreased libido and impotence. It is not known if these effects are a consequence of the depression that often accompanies methylmercury poisoning (Schragg & Dixon, 1985).

Mercury vapour

The potential adverse effects of mercury vapour on fertility is the subject of much current interest. Mercury vapour is much more readily absorbed than ingested mercury. Animal experiments have shown reduced fertility in rodents chronically exposed to inorganic mercury. Studies in Eastern Europe of workers exposed to mercury have shown menstrual disturbances including alterations in cycle length which may presumably be secondary to hormonal effects (Rowland *et al.*, 1994). One recent report describes the presence of mercury grains within the Leydig cells of a man with azoospermia and testicular atrophy who had been occupationally exposed to mercury vapour for 5 years (Keck *et al.*, 1993).

Mercury is the main component of amalgams used for filling dental cavities. Amalgams give off mercury vapour and this accounts for betwen 50% and 70% of the total mercury retained by non-occupationally exposed humans. This increases significantly when multiple fillings are inserted or removed. Dental assistants who make the almalgams are particularly exposed. A recent epidemiological survey of over 400 dental assistants found that those who prepared 30 or more dental amalgams per week associated with poor mercury hygiene factors had a per cycle conception rate of only 63% of that of unexposed dental assistants (Rowland *et al.*, 1994). This study was controlled for many confounding variables such as age, frequency of intercourse, number of sexual partners, etc.

Other metals

Cadmium

Cadmium is used in electroplating, manufacturing of plastics and batteries and in paints. It is also present in high concentrations in shellfish and cigarettes. Data on antifertility effects are inconclusive. In animals exposed to cadmium, ovarian toxicity has been demonstrated in the form of inhibition of ovulation, oocyte chromosome abnormalities and ovarian haemorrhage. It appears that the toxicity may be secondary to vascular damage. There are no human data implicating cadmium in infertility.

Animal data in males show testicular damage as a consequence of vascular disruption of the microcirculation of the testes. One autopsy study in a small group of four men involved in the production of cadmium-containing batteries showed no spermatids or only occasional spermatozoa in the testes. However, mitosis was still occurring within spermatocytes so the conclusions are not clear. Other studies have found no increase in infertility in cadmium-exposed workers, although in unexposed men there is a moderate correlation between cadmium levels in seminal plasma and sperm motility and velocity (Schragg & Dixon, 1985; Miller & Bellinger, 1994).

Manganese

Manganese is a weak reproductive toxicant. A report published in the 1950s described a small group of Chilean miners exposed to manganese, with decreased libido and difficulty ejaculating in approximately 25%. A more recent questionnaire in workers exposed to manganese dust revealed a significant reduction in the number of children born during the period of exposure (Lauwerys *et al.*, 1985).

Organic solvents

Solvents are substances that dissolve other substances. Over 30 000 industrial solvents have been classified. The absorption of the solvent depends on its physical and chemical properties, but common routes are via the skin and by inhalation. Several organic solvents have been implicated in reproductive disorders.

Ethylene glycol ethers

Over 100 glycol ethers are available. They are used in deicing fluids, in photography, electronics, painting and cleaning industries amongst others. The two most studied ethers are 2-methoxyethanol (2-ME) and 2-ethoxyethanol (2-EE). In animal experiments, these have been shown to lead to infertility, abnormal sperm morphology, degeneration of seminiferous epithelium and testicular atrophy at doses similar to those found in a workplace environment. Several studies have looked at reproductive effects in men exposed to ethylene glycol. The earliest in 1982 studied men working in an ethylene glycol production plant and found decreased testicular size but no sperm abnormality. Men who used glycol ethers as part of a slurry in a foundry had reduced sperm counts. A study of shipyard painters in 1988 showed a higher incidence of oligozoospermia and azoospermia in exposed workers (Welch *et al.*, 1988). Ethylene glycol is metabolised in the body to ethoxyacetic acid (EAA) and methoxyacetic acid (MAA). A recent case controlled study showed that the risk of infertility was three times greater in couples where the male had measurable EAA and MAA in the urine (Veulemans *et al.*, 1993). There are no reports of occupational exposure to ethylene glycol in women.

Carbon disulphide

The main use of carbon disulphide is in the production of viscose rayon. Studies in Romania, Italy and Finland in the 1970s suggested that chronic exposure over years is associated with reduced sperm parameters, altered gonadotrophin levels and decreased libido. Dose-response relationships have not been identified. A subsequent study in the USA in men exposed over several months showed no difference between exposed individuals and controls (Schragg & Dixon, 1985).

A controlled study investigated 116 men occupationally exposed to carbon disulphide compared with 79 non-exposed workers. The exposed group had significant reductions in libido and potency but there was no difference in the sperm parameters or fertility between the two groups (Vanhoorne, Comhaire & De Bacquer, 1994).

Other solvents

Several reports from Eastern Europe in the 1960s and 1970s described menstrual disorders in women working with toluene, benzene, xylene, styrene, carbon disulphide and formaldehyde. Little information is available on the dose of exposure or on other potential confounding variables. A large study in the USA in 1500 workers exposed to styrene found no increased incidence of menstrual abnormality (Welch, 1994).

Conflicting reports have appeared describing reduced sperm counts in males exposed to dinitrotoluene and toluene in a plant in Kentucky, but no abnormalities of count, morphology, FSH levels or reproductive history in a sister plant in Louisiana (Schragg & Dixon, 1985). A recent report from China, where workers were exposed to high concentrations of trinitrotoluene, found loss of libido and impotence in the exposed workers compared with controls. Semen parameters were also affected with reduced volume of seminal plasma, lower sperm motility and an increased percentage of abnormal forms. Serum testosterone levels were lower in exposed workers (Li *et al.*, 1993).

Pesticides

Nothing illustrates the potential reproductive problems caused by environmental toxicants as well as the pesticides. In the USA for example, 729 active ingredients and 1200 inert ingredients are used in 21 000 registered pesticide products. Pesticides are used in commercial agriculture and domestic gardening, in pest control and insect repellants. Treated agricultural land drains into rivers that feed the reservoirs that provide drinking water. Fruits and vegetables are sprayed with pesticide products. In the UK before the 1980s, the use of pesticides was overseen by voluntary schemes which depended on the close cooperation of the pesticide industry. It is not now possible to be sure which products were in use before that time. Since 1986, the Control of Pesticide regulations only allow the use of pesticides that have been sanctioned by the ministers of six government departments!

Dibromochloropropane (DBCP)

The first reports of fertility problems related to pesticides only appeared in 1977 when five men working at the manufacturing plant producing DBCP reported that they had not recently fathered children and were found to have severely reduced sperm counts or azoospermia. Following on from this report, a larger study was performed in 142 non-vasectomised men of whom 107 had been exposed to DBCP. There was a significant difference in sperm counts between exposed and non-exposed men: 30% of exposed men were azoospermic or severely oligozoospermic compared with 3% of controls (Whorton *et al.*, 1979). DBCP appears to lead to atrophy of the seminiferous epithelium in the most severely affected cases, although the effect of DBCP may be reversible if the degree of impaired spermatogenesis is not too severe. Reversibility is related to the duration of exposure and is more likely if FSH levels are not raised (Shragg & Dixon, 1985).

Although DBCP was banned in the USA in 1979, its repercussions are still significant. In Costa Rica it was reported that 1500 workers became sterile following exposure to DBCP in large commercial banana plantations and several hundred of these have filed law suits against the manufacturers (Thrupp, 1991).

Ethylene dibromide (EDB)

A retrospective investigation in 1979 studied the ratio of expected to observed births in couples in whom the male was occupationally exposed to EDB. In one of the four plants assessed, there were significantly less births than expected (Wong *et al.*, 1979). A subsequent study of men in the papaya fumigation industry in Hawaii showed that, in comparison to unexposed controls, the exposed men showed significantly reduced sperm density and motility and a higher percentage of sperm morphological abnormalities (Ratcliffe *et al.*, 1987). These findings have been confirmed in other studies, which have also shown reduced semen volume and increased semen pH, suggesting an effect on the accessory sex glands

(Schrader, Turner and Ratcliffe, 1988). Although EDB was banned from agricultural use in the USA in 1984, it is still in use as an anti-knock additive in lead-free petrol.

Chloredecone (kepone)

Following a severe poisoning incident in a manufacturing plant in 1975 workers exposed to chloredecone developed a serious clinical disorder resulting from central nervous system effects and oligozoospermia, with many immotile and abnormally formed sperm. In the worst affected cases, evidence of damage to the seminiferous epithelium was found on testicular biopsy (Moses, 1994). In 13 patients, the elimination of chloredecone was hastened by administering cholestyramine and it was noted that the number of motile sperm increased as serum chloredecone levels reduced (Schragg & Dixon, 1985). This would suggest a dose-related effect.

Other pesticides

In a recent study of over 1000 male Indian cotton workers exposed to pesticides, fewer live births were recorded compared with a non-exposed control group. In this study the effect was greater in exposed men who smoked (Rupa, Reddy & Reddi, 1991).

Concern has been expressed about other pesticides such as 2,4,5-trichlorophenoxyacetic acid (2,4,5-T), which is of relatively low toxicity but is contaminated with toxic breakdown products called dioxins. One survey found fewer conceptions in the wives of employees at a manufacturing plant who were exposed to dioxins than in the wives of non-exposed employees (Moses, 1994). DDT was extensively used at the end of the Second World War to destroy lice responsible for the spread of typhoid. It was also used to control mosquitoes and household flies. DDT has not been used in developed countries since the early 1970s when it became apparent that it accumulates in the environment and is harmful to animal life. It is still used in significant quantites in developing countries (Sharp, 1995). Recent evidence suggests that DDT may be responsible for a reduction in sperm counts in men (see p. 144).

Polyhalogenated biphenyls

Polyhalogenated biphenyls are halogenated aromatic hydrocarbons that are very resistant to degradation and persist for many years in the environment. Two types of these compound have been particularly studied for adverse reproductive effects.

Polychlorinated biphenyls (PCBs)

The PCBs permeate the environment. Although now banned, they were extensively used as fluids in transformers and capacitors as well as being used in the manufacture of plastics, carbonless copy paper and paints. They are present throughout the food chain and are ubiquitous in breast milk. They have also been found in ovarian follicular fluid. In studies in rodents involving administration of high concentrations of PCB, fertility was reduced in males, and this was associated with sperm disorders. In female animals, ovulatory disturbances are associated with reduced fertility (Paul, 1994b). PCBs may act by inducing hepatic enzymes responsible for the synthesis of sex hormone-binding globulin. They also have a weak oestrogen-like effect. No fertility studies have been performed in humans related to PCB exposure although PCB concentrations were similar in one study of semen from fertile and non-fertile men. In one small investigation involving *in vitro* fertilisation, semen samples that successfully fertilised oocytes and led to pregnancy contained a lower average concentration of PCB than those samples where the outcome of *in vitro* fertilisation was unsuccessful (as well as lower levels of other chemicals including hexachlorobenzene). Recent work has also shown that PCBs are present in higher concentration in cervical mucus than in blood and appear to reduce sperm motility in the mucus (Feichtinger, 1991).

Polybrominated biphenyls (PBBs)

The PBBs differ from PCBs only by the substitution of bromine for chlorine. They have similar resistance to degradation but had a limited production compared with PCB. They were mainly used as fire retardants in plastics. Accidental human exposure occurred in 1973–4 following inadvertent administration of a PBB-based product to thousands of cattle in Michigan as agricultural feed. Farm workers and consumers of meat in the area were, therefore, exposed. No adverse health effects have been recorded. The results of reproductive experiments in which rodents were fed PBB are similar to those for PCB. Data on human farm workers exposed to PBB showed no difference in sperm parameters 4 years after exposure compared with non-exposed controls. There was no correlation between PBB level and sperm concentration or testosterone levels. However, as the studies were performed several years after the incident, it is not known whether recovery had already occurred (Schragg & Dixon 1985; Paul, 1994b).

Occupational exposure to therapeutic agents

Several therapeutic drugs are known to affect male and/or female reproductive performance. These effects are discussed in the appropriate chapters. However the manufacture of these compounds may involve chronic occupational exposure for workers in the pharmaceutical industry. The main areas where problems have arisen are with the sex hormones. In addition, health care workers may be chronically exposed to drugs or chemicals used in patient treatment. Nurses or pharmacists involved in the preparation of antineoplastic drugs are at particular risk of accidental contamination. The case of mercury vapour exposure in dental assistants has been described earlier in this chapter. Much current concern is focused on the occupational risks in both anaesthetists and others who use nitrous oxide inhalational anaesthesia.

Sex steroids

Workers at a factory in Puerto Rico that formulated synthetic oestrogen and progestogen contraceptive pills were investigated and it was shown that 20% of males experienced symptoms related to hyperoestrogenism, including gynaecomastia. Some also had reduced libido or impotence. Plasma ethinyloestradiol levels were raised. Women in the plant were four times more likely than controls to experience intermenstrual bleeding (Harrington *et al.*, 1978). Hyperoestrogenism has also been reported in workers, and their children, in a Polish plant manufacturing diethylstilboestrol (Schragg & Dixon, 1985). It is possible to eliminate this risk virtually completely in modern contraceptive pill manufacturing facilities by efficient dust extraction systems and protective clothing (McDiarmid, 1994).

Antineoplastics

The antineoplastic drugs are known to have significant antifertility effects (see Chapter 4). Current practice in pharmaceutical plants manufacturing these agents has minimised occupational exposure to workers. The major risk of exposure is by skin contact or inhalation during the preparation and administration of these drugs by doctors, nurses and pharmacists. Studies of occupational exposure to date have concentrated on the risks of pregnancy loss or fetal abnormality. However, as these drugs have marked antifertility effects in cancer patients, it is likely that reproductive capacity may be compromised following exposure. It is suggested that exposed personnel delay attempts at conception for 3 months. The Occupational Safety and Health Administration in the USA recommends that male and female workers who are trying to conceive, are pregnant or are breast feeding, should be offered alternative duties that do not involve handling antineoplastics (McDiarmid, 1994).

Anaesthetic gases

Nitrous oxide

Many studies have been performed since the 1970s looking at reproductive risks associated with anaesthetic gases and particularly nitrous oxide (N_2O) in operating room personnel. Several studies linked N_2O exposure to spontaneous abortion and an increased risk of congenital abnormality. Two studies reported decreased fertility in women exposed to mixed anaesthetic gases. Many of these studies have been criticised for several reasons, including few data and lack of accounting for confounding variables. Anaesthetists and operating room personnel are more informed about health risks than most occupationally exposed workers and this could also bias results. A recent important paper has now renewed interest in the potential danger of N_2O to health workers (Rowland *et al.*, 1992). This study assessed the number of cycles necessary to achieve a pregnancy related to the level of exposure of female dental assistants to N_2O. The most significant result was that women exposed to N_2O without scavenging equipment for more than 5 hours per week had a 60% reduction in their chances of conception each month. The same amount of exposure to N_2O when scavenging equipment was used was not associated with reduced fertility, demonstrating the importance of protective measures. The National Institute for Occupational Safety and Health in the USA recommend a standard of 25 p.p.m. for N_2O, although the mean levels of exposure in 20 dental surgeries surveyed was greater than 100 p.p.m. (Baird, 1992). In animal studies, fertility is reduced at doses of approximately 500 p.p.m.

Although a study as early as 1971 suggested a history of infertility in males exposed to N_2O the Rowland paper has rekindled awareness of these potential adverse effects (Baird, 1992).

Two mechanisms have been proposed whereby N_2O might impair fertility. In rats, it blocks the secretion of GnRH from the hypothalamus, which prevents ovulation. N_2O also oxidises vitamin B_{12} and inactivates the vitamin B_{12}-dependent enzyme methionine synthetase. This is involved in DNA synthesis and hence may interrupt cell mitosis in rapidly dividing cells such as the spermatogenic cells in men and ovarian granulosa cells in women.

Are men becoming less fertile?

A paper published in 1992 generated enormous interest in the scientific press as well as in the lay media in the possibility that some unknown environmental factor was causing a significant decline in human sperm counts.

The authors performed a literature review and identified 61 papers published between 1938 and 1990 that included data on a total of 14 947 men. Papers dealing with men with fertility problems were excluded. Details of sperm density and semen volume were recorded. Between 1940 and 1990 the mean seminal volume decreased from 3.40 to 2.75 ml. The mean semen concentration decreased from 113×10^6/ml to 66×10^6/ml. Both these results represent statistically significant decreases. This, coupled with reports of increased male genitourinary abnormalities over the years, led the authors to conclude that the changes were more likely to be caused by environmental rather than genetic factors (Carlsen *et al.*, 1992).

The conclusions of this paper cannot be ignored, although there has been considerable controversy over the interpretation of the results. For example, only 13 of the 61 studies were performed before 1970. Reanalysis of the data in the remaining 48 papers since 1970 by other scientists has shown that there has been no decline in sperm concentration since that time. If anything there has been a small increase (Brake & Krause, 1992). Furthermore, assessment of sperm counts is subjective and reproducibility is poor. It is difficult to be certain that results from 1938 in one country can be compared with those in 1990 in another.

Measurements of semen volumes are more accurate and reproducible and a clear reduction has been demonstrated. However, the volume of ejaculate depends on the period of sexual abstinence. This was not assessed in the analysis of results. The authors simply conclude that there are no data to suggest that there has been a change in the frequency of ejaculation since the 1930s and, therefore, presumably they do not believe the period of abstinence to be responsible for the decline.

Some of these uncertainties have been addressed by a recent publication from Paris which looked at the semen characteristics of 1351 fertile sperm donors assessed in a single laboratory over a 20-year period using standardised methodology. The authors demonstrated that, over this time period, there had been a reduction in sperm count by 2.1% per year, and a reduction of sperm motility and morphology by 0.6% and 0.5% per year, respectively. In this analysis, they were able to control for the age of the man and the period of sexual abstinence. The reduction in sperm quality was still apparent even after these factors were excluded. No change was reported in the semen volume, although these authors used seminal plasma weight as an estimation of semen volume (Auger *et al.*, 1995).

Role of environmental oestrogens

In 1993 another paper published in the Lancet attracted much media interest (Sharpe & Skakkebæck, 1993). The authors noted that the reduction in sperm counts over the past 50 years has been paralleled by an increase in disorders of the male reproductive tract in a similar time frame. In particular the incidence of testicular cancer, testicular maldescent (cryptorchidism) and urethral abnormalities (hypospadias) have risen. Male fetuses of women exposed to DES showed a high incidence of cryptorchidism and hypospadias as well as a possible increased incidence of testicular cancer. By tying these two observations together, Sharpe and Skakkebæck reasoned that environmental oestrogens may be responsible for both phenomena. They postulate that male fetuses are exposed to higher concentrations of oestrogens during intrauterine life than was the case 50 years ago, accounting for both reduced sperm numbers and the increased incidence of genital tract abnormailities.

Suggested sources of oestrogens are both endogenous and exogenous. Absorption of synthetic oestrogens may result from the use of oral contraceptives, which are excreted and may be recycled into drinking water. Natural oestrogens may be ingested from plants rich in oestrogens such as soya, and increased consumption of dairy product such as cow's milk which contains oestrogens. Many chemicals found in the environment, such as PCB and dioxin, also have oestrogenic activity.

This is all supposition, but data from lakes that have been polluted with oestrogenic chemicals add some weight to the hypothesis. A spill of the pesticide DDT into a lake in Florida in 1980 has been associated with a 90% decline in the birthrate of alligators and a reduction in the size of the penis in many of the young alligators. Male fish have shown features of feminisation in other polluted waters (Anon., 1994). Protagonists of the reproductive hazards of environmental oestrogens point to this and other wildlife data as stark evidence of the link between oestrogens and reproductive disorders. Opponents, however, claim it is inappropriate to compare the results following a massive episode of poisoning with the relatively small amount of exposure to which the average human is exposed. The oestrogen hypothesis will undoubtedly continue to occupy the minds of reproductive scientists and the lay public for some time to come.

A potentially significant development in this story is the recent discovery that the major metabolite of the pesticide DDT is a potent androgen antagonist. Kelce and co-workers in a series of experiments in rats have shown that *p,p'*-DDE is an androgen receptor antagonist that has the same degree of activity as powerful antiandrogens (Kelce *et al.,* 1995). They suggest that the reproductive tract abnormalities reported in animals and humans, which had previously been linked to environmental oestrogenic chemicals, may be caused by this compound. By preventing normal androgenic action, it exerts a demasculinising rather than a feminising effect.

p,p'-DDE interfered with the male reproductive tract at all stages in development. The male offspring of pregnant rats exposed to *p,p'*-DDE had reproductive tract abnormalities at birth. Immature male rats treated with this compound experienced delay in the onset of puberty. When given to mature rats, p,p'-DDE reduced the weight of the seminal vesicle and prostate gland.

The amount of *p,p'*-DDE necessary to exert antiandrogenic effects *in vitro* was 64 parts per billion (p.p.b.). Following the DDT spill in Lake Apopka in Florida described above, the eggs of the demasculinised alligators contained 5800 p.b.b. When DDT was still in use in the USA in the 1960s, levels of 650–3750 p.p.b. were found in the tissues of stillborn babies (Kelce *et al.,* 1995).

DDT is now not used in the developed world but as it has a halflife of 100 years it is ubiquitous in humans, where it is stored in body fat. Furthermore, it is still used in vast quantities in Mexico and Brazil and by accumulation in the food chain can be transmitted to countries where its use is proscribed (Sharpe, 1995). If *p,p'*-DDE is related to declining sperm quality in males, this problem may well persist for several generations.

References

Anon (1994). Environmental estrogens stir debate. *Science,* 265, 308–10.
Auger, J., Kunstmann, J. M. Czyglik, F. & Jouannet, P. (1995) Decline in semen quality among fertile men in Paris during the past 20 years. *New England Journal of Medicine,* 332, 281–5.
Baird, P. A. (1992). Occupational exposure to nitrous oxide–not a laughing matter. *New England Journal of Medicine,* 327, 1026–7.
Baranski, B. (1993). Effects of the workplace on fertility and related reproductive outcomes. *Environmental Health Perspective,* 101 (suppl 2), 81–90.
Brake, A. & Krause, W. (1992). Decreasing quality of semen. *British Medical Journal,* 305, 1948.

Brent. R., Meistrich, M. & Paul, M. (1994). Ionising and non ionising radiations. In *Occupational and Environmetal Reproductive Hazards*, ed. M. Paul, pp. 165–89. Baltimore: Williams and Wilkins.

Carlsen, E., Giwercman, A., Keiding, N. & Skakkebæk, N.E. (1992). Evidence for decreasing quality of semen during the past 50 years. *British Medical Journal*, 305, 609–16.

Feichtinger, W. (1991). Environmental factors and fertility. *Human Reproduction*, 6, 1170–5 .

Harrington, J. M., Stein, G. F., Rivera, R. O. & de Morales, A. V. (1978). The occupational hazards of formulating oral contraceptives: a survey of plant employees. *Archives of Environmental Health*, 33, 12–15.

Hughes, S. (1993). Radiation exposure in the UK. *Radiological Protection Bulletin*, 145, 10–12.

Keck, C., Bergmann, M., Ernst, E., Muller, C., Kliesch, S. & Nieschlag, E. (1993). Autometallographic detection of mercury in testicular tissue of an infertile man exposed to mercury vapor. *Reproductive Toxicology*, 7, 469–75.

Kelce, W. R., Stone, C. R., Laws S. C., Earl Gray, L., Kemppainen, J. A. & Wilson, E. M. (1995). Persistent DDT metabolite p,p′-DDE is a potent androgen receptor antagonist.*Nature*, 375, 581–5.

Lauwerys, R., Roels, H., Genet, P., Toussaint, G., Bouckaert, A. & De Cooman, S. (1985). Fertility of male workers exposed to mercury vapour or to manganese dust: a questionnaire survey. *American Journal of Industrial Medicine*, 7, 171–6.

Li, Y., Jiang, Q. G., Yao, S. Q., Liu, W., Tian, G. J. & Cui, J. W. (1993). Effects of exposure to trinitrotoluene on male reproduction. *Biomedical and Environmental Sciences*, 6, 154–60.

Mattison, D. R. & Thomford, P. J. (1989). The mechanisms of action of reproductive toxicants. *Toxicologic Pathology*, 17, 364–76.

McDiarmid, M. (1994). Occupational exposure to pharmaceuticals: antineoplastics, anaesthetics agents, sex steroid hormones. In *Occupational and Environmental Reproductive Hazards*, ed. M. Paul, pp. 280–95. Baltimore: Williams and Wilkins.

Miller, R. K. & Bellinger, D. (1994).Metals. In *Occupational and Environmental Reproductive Hazards*, ed. M. Paul, pp. 233–52. Baltimore: Williams and Wilkins.

Moses, M. (1994). Pesticides. In *Occupational and Environmental Reproductive Hazards*, ed. M. Paul, pp. 296–309. Baltimore: Williams and Wilkins.

National Radiation Protection Board (1994). Radiation Protection Standards. Didcot, Oxon, U.K. National Radiation Protection Board.

Paul, M. (ed.) (1994a). *Occupational and Environmental Reproductive Hazards*. Baltimore: Williams and Wilkins.

Paul, M. (1994b). Polyhalogenated biphenyls. In *Occupational and Environmental Reproductive Hazards*. ed. M. Paul, pp. 310–18. Baltimore: Williams and Wilkins.

Plowchalk, D., Meadows, M. J. & Mattison D. R. (1994). Female reproductive toxicology. In *Occupational and Environmental Reproductive Hazards*, ed. M. Paul, pp. 18–24. Baltimore: Williams and Wilkins.

Ratcliffe, J. M., Schrader, S. M., Steenland, K., Clapp, D. E., Turner, T. & Hornung, R. W. (1987). Semen quality in papaya workers with long term exposure to ethylene dibromide. *British Journal of Industrial Medicine*, 44, 317–26.

Rowland, A. S., Baird, D. D., Weinberg, C. R., Shore, D. L., Shy, C. M. & Wilcox, A. J. (1992). Reduced fertility among women employed as dental assistants exposed to high levels of nitrous oxide. *New England Journal of Medicine*, 327, 993–7.

Rowland, A. S., Baird, D. D., Weinberg, C. R., Shore, D. L., Shy, C. M. & Wilcox, A. J. (1994) The effect of occupational exposure to mercury vapour on the fertility of female dental assistants. *Occupational and Environmental Medicine*, 51, 28–34.

Rupa, D. S., Reddy, P. P. & Reddi, O. S. (1991). Reproductive performance in population exposed to pesticides in cotton fields in India. *Environmental Research*, 55, 123–8.

Schrader, S. M. & Kesner, J. S. (1994). Male reproductive toxicology. In *Occupational and Environmental Reproductive Hazards*, ed. M. Paul, pp. 3–17. Baltimore: Williams and Wilkins.

Schrader, S. M., Turner, T. W. & Ratcliffe, J. M. (1988). The effects of ethylene dibromide on semen quality: a comparison of short-term and chronic exposure. *Reproductive Toxicology*, 2, 191–8.

Schragg, S. D. & Dixon, R. L. (1985). Occupational exposures associated with male reproductive dysfunction. *Annual Review of Pharmacology and Toxicology*, 25, 567–92.

Scialli, A. R. (1992). Advances in reproductive toxicology. *Current Opinion in Obstetrics and Gynecology*, 4, 359–64.

Sharpe, R. M. (1995). Another DDT connection . *Nature*, 375, 538–9.

Sharpe, R. M. & Skakkebæk, N. E. (1993). Are oestrogens involved in falling sperm counts and disorders of the male reproductive tract? *Lancet*, 341, 1392–5.

Thrupp, L. A. (1991). Sterilisation of workers from pesticide exposure: the causes and consequences of DBCP-induced damage in Costa Rica and beyond. *International Journal of Health Services*, 21, 731–57.

Vanhoorne, M., Comhaire, F. & De Bacquer, D. (1994). Epidemiological study of the effects of carbon disulfide on male sexuality and reproduction. *Archives of Environmental Health*, 49, 273–8.

Veulemans, H., Steeno, O., Masschelein, R. & Groeseneken, D. (1993). Exposure to ethylene glycol ethers and spermatogenic disorders in man: a case control study. *British Journal of Industrial Medicine*, 50, 71–8.

Welch, L. S. (1994). Organic solvents. In *Occupational and Environmental Reproductive Hazards*, ed. M. Paul, pp. 267–79. Baltimore: Williams and Wilkins.

Welch, L. S., Schrader, S. M., Turner, T. W. & Cullen, M. R. (1988). Effects of exposure to ethylene glycol esters on shipyard painters: II. Male reproduction. *American Journal of Industrial Medicine*, 14, 509–26.

Whorton, D., Milby, T. H., Krauss, R. M. & Stubbs, H. A. (1979). Testicular function in DBCP exposed pesticide workers. *Journal of Occupational Medicine*, 21, 161–6.

Wong, O,. Utidjian, H. M. & Karten, V. S. (1979). *Journal of Occupational Medicine*, 21, 98–102.

Index